Asperger's Syndrome and Sexuality

of related interest

Asperger's Syndrome
A Guide for Parents and Professionals
Tony Attwood
Foreword by Lorna Wing
ISBN 1 85302 577 1

Asperger Syndrome in Adolescence
Living with the Ups, the Downs and Things in Between
Edited by Liane Holliday Willey
Foreword by Luke Jackson
ISBN 1 84310 742 2

Freaks, Geeks and Asperger Syndrome
A User Guide to Adolescence
Luke Jackson
Foreword by Tony Attwood
ISBN 1 84310 098 3

Pretending to be Normal
Living with Asperger's Syndrome
Liane Holliday Willey
Foreword by Tony Attwood
ISBN 1 85302 749 9

Asperger Syndrome and Long-Term Relationships
Ashley Stanford
Foreword by Liane Holliday Willey
ISBN 1 84310 734 1

Aspergers in Love
Couple Relationships and Family Affairs
Maxine Aston
Foreword by Gisela and Chris Slater-Walker
ISBN 1 84310 115 7

Sex, Sexuality and the Autism Spectrum
Wendy Lawson
Foreword by Glenys Jones
ISBN 1 84310 284 6

Asperger's Syndrome and Sexuality

From Adolescence through Adulthood

Isabelle Hénault

Foreword by Tony Attwood

Jessica Kingsley Publishers
London and Philadelphia

First published in 2006
by Jessica Kingsley Publishers
116 Pentonville Road
London N1 9JB, UK
and
400 Market Street, Suite 400
Philadelphia, PA 19106, USA
www.jkp.com

Copyright © Isabelle Hénault 2006
Foreword copyright © Tony Attwood 2006
Translation by Julie Larouche
Front cover photograph by Amélie Bolduc-Monette

Library of Congress Cataloging in Publication Data

Hénault, Isabelle, 1973-
    Asperger's syndrome and sexuality : from adolescence through adulthood / Isabelle Hénault ; foreword by Tony
Attwood.— 1st American pbk. ed.
        p. cm.
    Includes bibliographical references and index.
    ISBN-13: 978-1-84310-189-5 (pbk. : alk. paper)
    ISBN-10: 1-84310-189-0 (pbk. : alk. paper) 1. Asperger's syndrome. 2. Autism. I. Title.
    RC553.A88H46 2006
    618.92'858832—dc22

                                                    2005024310

British Library Cataloguing in Publication Data

A CIP catalogue record for this book is available from the British Library

ISBN-13: 978 1 84310 189 5
ISBN-10: 1 84310 189 0

Printed and Bound in Great Britain by
Athenaeum Press, Gateshead, Tyne and Wear

Contents

LIST OF FIGURES, BOXES AND TABLES

Acknowledgements

My greatest respect goes to Dr Tony Attwood for his inspiration and generosity; he has made it possible for me to fulfil my greatest dreams. A special thank you to Julie Larouche for her professionalism and her friendship that is so dear to me. Thanks go to Jessica for her confidence in me and her patience throughout the realization of this project. I would also like to express my gratitude to my parents, Jean and Jeanne, and to my sister, Geneviève. They have supported and encouraged me to pursue my path from the very beginning. They never ceased to believe that everything is possible. All my gratitude goes to Charles, my love. His involvement has been extraordinary and so motivating. His encouraging comments and humour were a great help during the writing of this book. A very special thank you goes to you, Charles. I am grateful to Georges, Marc-Antoine, Stef, Martine, Ron, and all the individuals with Asperger's Syndrome who agreed to broach such a personal and sensitive topic with such sincerity and openness. My thanks also extend to Lise Durocher and Martine Fortier for permission to adapt activities from their sexual education programme, to Patrick Papazian for ideas and collaboration, and Amélie Bolduc-Monette for her photographic savvy. Finally, I would like to acknowledge Dr Normand Giroux, who introduced me to this area and who has continued to guide me over the last six years. I dedicate this book to him.

Foreword

People with Asperger's Syndrome (AS) have the same sexual interests, issues and diversity as occur in the general population. However, adolescents and adults with AS are different in terms of the ability to 'read' and understand the subtle and complex thoughts and emotions of another person and to effectively communicate their own inner thoughts and feelings. There are also differences in sensory perception, previous relationship experiences and the understanding of social conventions. These differences are obviously going to have a significant impact on the development of sexuality for the person with AS. While we are gradually increasing our knowledge base and expertise on AS, there is a separate and extensive knowledge base and expertise on sexuality in the general population. What has been missing is someone with qualifications and clinical expertise in both areas to combine an understanding of AS and sexuality and to write the seminal book on sexual education and intervention programmes. Isabelle Hénault has now written that book.

The author first provides factual information on the physiological and psychological changes associated with puberty, the development of intimate relationships and the range of human sexuality that is relevant to adolescents and adults with AS. People with AS enjoy increasing their knowledge and acquiring and remembering facts, but the area of sexuality is more than a collection of facts and data. There are issues of self-perception and self-esteem, attitudes and prejudices, past experiences, empathy and intimacy. Isabelle Hénault takes a broad perspective of sexuality and applies her extensive and intuitive knowledge of AS to develop effective sexual education programmes that will improve the quality of life and relationships, not only of people with AS but also those who develop an intimate relationship with them. Not only will psychologists and educators implement the programmes developed and evaluated by Isabelle Hénault, but the parents, friends and partners of people with AS will also find the information and strategies in *Asperger's Syndrome and Sexuality* of considerable interest.

People with AS will also benefit from reading this book, developing a greater understanding of their own sexuality and improving their ability to achieve and maintain a successful intimate relationship. It is essential that in the quest for knowledge on sexuality, a person (especially someone with AS), has access to correct and appropriate information. An adolescent with AS may assume that his or her peer group has reliable knowledge about sexuality, due to their willingness to discuss sexual matters openly and frequently. They are the apparent experts. Unfortunately, the adolescent peer group may not be the most knowledgeable source of information and some typical adolescents may enjoy the opportunity to misinform someone with AS who seems naïve and gullible. This book is a source of accurate and reassuring information, as well as providing practical advice. If you are someone with AS or care for someone with AS, this book will be read and referred to many times. Be careful with regard to whom you lend it, as they may be reluctant to return it.

Tony Attwood, author of the bestselling book
Asperger's Syndrome: A Guide for Parents and Professionals

Introduction

I got the idea for writing a book on the sexuality of individuals with Asperger's Syndrome (AS) during my doctoral studies. After consulting a broad range of scientific literature, I found, to my great surprise, that only three publications dealt with the sexuality of individuals with autism. How could this be explained? Preconceived notions, taboos, and lack of data were all too evident. How could such a universal topic be ignored, especially since AS has been recognized in the DSM-IV since 1994 (APA 1994)? The literature that does exist tends to address aetiological factors (genetic, environmental, neuro-chemical, etc.); treatment strategies are largely ignored.

Information on the sexuality of individuals with AS is lacking in current scientific literature. However, despite the superficial resistance that accompanies the exploration of sexuality, individuals with AS have been open-minded and curious about the topic. Issues related to their needs need to be explored in order to identify the types of intervention required to ensure their well-being, sexual health, and sexual education. Individuals with AS have the same interests and sexual needs as the general population; however, their mode of expression is different. Their communication difficulties add to the obstacles that they encounter when establishing interpersonal and sexual relationships. The purpose of this book is to offer guidance on sexual development, behaviour, relationships, and education, adapted to the needs of individuals of all ages living with AS.

Sexuality is, happily, an unavoidable reality. Humans explore their sexuality in a variety of ways, at all stages of development. The discovery of one's body, pleasure, the opposite sex, the forbidden and so on, usually takes place without any major obstacles. However, sexuality can be quite different for someone with AS. Personal characteristics, circumscribed interests, sensory sensitivity, world view, and interpersonal difficulties can all be problematic. The sexual reality of someone with AS usually goes unnoticed and is frequently repressed, misunderstood, and incorrectly interpreted. Nevertheless, by showing interest and offering people with AS simple and effective intervention strategies, we acknowledge that they are sexual beings too.

The aim of this book is to establish a positive perspective on sexuality and to defuse issues that are too often perceived as problematic behaviours or perversions. While these do occur in the Asperger population, sexuality here will be addressed more broadly: factors such as intimacy, friendship, desire, communication, gender, preferences, identity, needs, emotions, and development are all considered and themes relevant to adolescence and adulthood are addressed. The book is split into two parts: Part 1 explores sexuality and AS (details of each chapter can be found below), and Part 2 consists of the education programme for the development of sociosexual skills.

Chapter 1 deals with puberty, physiological changes, exploration of sexual behaviours, and self-esteem. A review of the literature in the field helps us to understand the factors related to the sexual development of individuals with AS.

Chapter 2 explores problematic sexual behaviours and factors that trigger inappropriate conduct or cause it to persist.

Chapter 3 addresses the topics of intimacy and communication with the aim of facilitating the communication of emotions. Emotions are at the core of interpersonal relationships and are discussed in great detail in order to provide a greater understanding of the different issues involved. Five rules of communication are presented and adapted to individuals with AS.

Chapter 4 addresses gender identity and sexual preferences. The possible relationship between gender identity and AS is receiving growing scientific attention, and clinical cases and Internet discussion groups provide examples of experimentation with different sexual roles, transvestitism, and transsexualism.

Chapter 5 examines couples, commitment, needs, partner expectations, and couple therapy. Personal testimonies of adults with AS are also presented, addressing topics such as intimacy, partnership, and sexuality.

Chapter 6 is an introduction to the sociosexual education programme in Part 2. The 12 workshops in the programme provide practical activities and tools, and include notes and detailed instructions for preparation. Each workshop deals with a specific topic.

The Appendix provides a sexual profile of adults with AS, based on a study conducted in collaboration with Dr Tony Attwood which compared the sexual profile of individuals with AS to that of the general population. Eleven aspects were explored (information, sexual desire, body image, behavioural repertoire, etc.) so as to better understand the reality of adults with AS.

A list of references, further reading, and resources can be found at the end of the book.

PART I

EXPLORING SEXUALITY AND ASPERGER'S SYNDROME

Chapter 1

Asperger's Syndrome and sexual development

Asperger's Syndrome

Individuals with Asperger's Syndrome (AS) experience a variety of problems related to social integration. Called upon to live in society, they need to be autonomous and show socially acceptable behaviours. Their lack of social ease is the major obstacle to effective integration into family and social circles. AS, a pervasive developmental disorder (PDD), was only recently recognized in the official nomenclature of the International Classification of Diseases (ICD-10; WHO, 1993) and in the DSM-IV (APA, 1994). Despite the ever-growing research attention that this complex disorder has received, the important issues of interpersonal relationships and sexuality remain neglected.

The syndrome was first described in a detailed manner in 1944 by Hans Asperger, an Austrian psychiatrist. His description of "autistic psychopathies" was based on observations of children in his clinic; his conclusions differed from those of Kanner (1943), who worked on autism. The scientific community first came to learn about the syndrome in 1981 from Lorna Wing's article "Asperger's Syndrome: A clinical account"; Asperger's original article was translated into English by Uta Frith in 1991.

Since 1998, clinicians and adults living with AS (Aston, 2001; Attwood, 1998a; Holliday Willey, 1999; Klin, Volkmar, and Sparrow, 2000) have become interested in helping individuals with AS, and a variety of practical works have become available. Attwood's (1998a) book *Asperger's Syndrome: A Guide for Parents and Professionals* is a key reference for all those interested or working in the field. Liane Holliday Willey has written two captivating autobiographical accounts of living with AS, *Pretending to be Normal* (1999) and *Asperger Syndrome in the Family: Redefining Normal* (2001). Her thoughts and commentary on the disorder are pertinent and very helpful for the lay public and professionals alike.

Current research attention is devoted to the prevalence of AS, diagnostic assessment, and intervention methods. Attwood's work (personal communication,

2002) shows a high prevalence of cases. He suggests a minimal prevalence of 0.20% (1 in 500) and a maximal prevalence of 0.50% (1 in 200), which is consistent with rates reported by Ehlers and Gillberg (1993). The male:female ratio is 4:1 and 10:1 in clinical settings (Attwood, 2002). These data show an increase in reported cases due to the recognition of the disorder by the World Health Organization (WHO) and by the American Psychiatric Association (APA), in addition to improved diagnostic criteria and techniques.

Asperger's Syndrome or high functioning autism?

There is considerable debate around the distinction between AS and high functioning autism. Some authors (e.g. Schopler, Mesibov, and Kunce, 1998) support the hypothesis that these two classifications belong to the same continuum of PDD. Others remain uncertain about the possibility of a significant difference between the two conditions (see Schopler *et al.*, 1998).

Attwood (2003b) believes that high functioning autism and AS are found on the same continuum. This view supports he use of intervention programmes for the whole autistic spectrum. Lorna Wing (1981) takes a similar view, noting that certain "classic" cases of autism progress to AS, especially if they receive early intervention.

Notwithstanding this debate, individuals with high functioning autism as well as those with AS present with specific difficulties in their sexual skills, and this book is addressed to both these populations.

There are at least four sets of diagnostic criteria for AS, including those in the ICD-10 (WHO, 1993), the DSM-IV (APA, 1994), those of Gillberg and Gillberg (1989), and those of Szatmari, Bremner and Nagy (1989), all of which are summarized below. To receive a diagnosis of AS, individuals must present with a number of characteristics of the Asperger profile.

Diagnostic criteria for Asperger's Syndrome

- No cognitive or language delay.

- Severe impairments in social interactions:
  - difficulty with visual contact, facial expression, nonverbal language
  - difficulty developing friendships
  - lack of emotional reciprocity
  - lack of empathy.

- Unusual, stereotyped, and restricted interests:
  - fixed routines and rituals
  - stereotyped behaviours and movements
  - intense interest in certain parts or aspects of objects (e.g. colour, texture).

- Impairment in social, occupational, and other important functioning.

- No delay in cognitive development; IQ greater than 70.

- Criteria are not met for another PDD, attachment disorder, obsessive compulsive disorder, or schizophrenia.

In addition to these formal criteria, the following clinical observations complete the diagnostic portrait:

- *Social isolation.* Individuals show a lack of interest in interpersonal relationships.

- *Communication.* Individuals do not decode nonverbal language cues, and verbal exchanges resemble a monologue rather than a two-way exchange. Neologisms (invented words) may be used.

- *Stereotyped gesticulations.* Tics, repetitive motor movements, etc.

- *Imagination and theory of mind.* Their level of cognitive development makes symbolic play possible, but individuals with AS experience deficits in relation to theory of mind. According to Tréhin (1999), theory of mind is defined as the capacity to attribute a mental state to oneself and others. This capacity for "meta-representation" is usually acquired at approximately four years of age, but its acquisition is delayed in the case of individuals with AS. The way they use their imagination is idiosyncratic: personal, original, and unique to the individual.

- *Sensory responses.* Hypo- and hypersensitivity of the senses. One sense is usually more developed than the others and serves as a reference point against which to assess the other senses.

- *Motor function.* Deficits in fine motor and hand–eye coordination skills as observed in body movements, gait, play, etc.

- *Emotions.* Individuals find them difficult to decode in themselves and in others.

- *Identity.* Lack of self-inquiry into social and sexual identity.

A number of questionnaires and diagnostic tools are available to formally assess characteristics of AS. The measures developed by Ehlers and Gillberg (1993) and the Australian Scale for Asperger's Syndrome (Garnett and Attwood, 1995, as cited in Attwood, 1998a) detect the presence of AS characteristics in children, whereas the Autism-Spectrum Quotient (Baron-Cohen *et al.*, 2001), and the Asperger Syndrome Diagnostic Scale (Smith Myles, Bock and Simpson, 2000) measure Asperger traits in adults.

Attwood and Gray (1999b) coined the term "Aspie" in their development of criteria aimed at measuring the strengths of individuals with AS. This positive approach, a significant departure from assessment procedures based on detecting deficits, is accompanied by intervention strategies that emphasize special abilities. The criteria can be summarized thus:

- Social interactions are based on authentic relationships with others. Individuals with AS are not judgemental, sexist, nor culturally biased in their interpersonal relationships.

- Language is developed and vocabulary is rich, but is often considered "pretentious".

- Cognitive abilities are characterized by attention to detail, and information is gathered on specific subjects.

- Individuals have a propensity for activities and hobbies that require endurance and concentration.

- Individuals possess encyclopaedic knowledge of specific subjects (for example aviation, insects, computers, history, numbers, calendars, etc.).

- Individuals may have an extraordinary long-term memory for facts and details: dates, names, schedules, routes .

- Some individuals are gifted in areas such as music, drawing, the sciences, etc.

There is little information on the clinical course of AS. Nonetheless, in theory, the appearance of symptoms allows for a diagnosis to be made from as early as three years of age. A child's differences are often noted very early on by parents, or by teaching staff during the first school years when increased contact with other children makes it possible to detect differential characteristics. AS constantly evolves over a person's lifetime. Behavioural interventions are of critical importance as they allow individuals to develop to their full potential and ameliorate specific difficulties.

Sexuality and Asperger's Syndrome

Despite the clear interest shown by several authors (e.g. Attwood, 1998a; Haracopos and Pedersen, 1999; Kempton, 1993; Klin *et al.*, 2000) in AS in general, few studies have examined specifically the sexual profile and skills of individuals living with the syndrome.

The tendency to define the sexuality of individuals as 'different' only serves to increase the resistance from others (parents, professionals, siblings, peers, etc.) and obstacles to the provision of the information and education that Aspies need. How often have researchers and professionals heard from parents and carers: "We have enough problems, don't talk to us about sexuality", or "If we talk to him about sexuality, he'll want to investigate it"?

In order to clear up these prejudices, here are five premises of the philosophy of adolescent and adult sexuality:

1. There is no positive correlation between knowledge of, and interest in, sexuality.

2. Adolescence is a period marked by curiosity and exploration; this phase of development is completely healthy.

3. Ignorance breeds fear (in the individual and his or her peer group). Information allows an individual with AS to develop their own judgement and puts them in a position to react better to a variety of situations.

4. A behaviour is less likely to be excessive if it is recognized, accepted, and appropriate in a given context, rather than forbidden.

5. Urges and sexual desires cannot be repressed; they must be directed towards appropriate expression.

Puberty

Several authors (e.g. Gillberg, 1983; Haracopos and Pedersen, 1999; Hellemans, 1996; Hingsburger, 1993; Ousley and Mesibov, 1991) consider the development of secondary sexual characteristics (hormonal increases, pilosity, genital maturation, etc.) in individuals with high functioning autism and AS comparable to that in the general population. In addition, these individuals demonstrate sociosexual interests and the same sexual needs as their peers. However, their communication difficulties and lack of social skills have an impact on their capacity and ability to engage in sexual interactions and increase the likelihood that inappropriate sexual behaviours will emerge.

The period of puberty takes place between the ages of 8 and 16 years and is associated with physiological changes related to the reproductive capacity of males and females. These characteristics can emerge in younger (precocious) or older (delayed) people with AS. Individual differences, family characteristics, and genetic factors play an important role in the timing of puberty. The process is usually complete between the ages of 18 and 22 years. This important milestone in sexual development is multifaceted, with changes occurring on the emotional, hormonal, social, interpersonal, and physiological fronts.

During adolescence, a number of issues need to be addressed. These constitute the basis of sexual education. Here are some examples (Sexuality Information and Education Council of the US, 1991):

- sexual organs of both sexes: names, functions, and concrete descriptions

- bodily changes that accompany puberty

- self-esteem, self-confidence, and body image

- nocturnal emissions and sexual cycle

- values and steps to decision-making, choices and maturity

- intimacy: private and public settings

- sexual health: behaviours and examination of male and female sexual organs

- dating, love, intimacy, and friendship

- how alcohol and drug use influence decision-making

- sexual intercourse and other sexual activities

- physical reactions, masturbation, and pleasure

- sexual orientation and identity

- birth control, menstruation, and hygiene

- condoms, contraception, and disease prevention

- emotions related to sexuality and interpersonal relationships.

Emotions related to sexuality should be included in discussions since they are likely to motivate many behaviours.

Guidance is essential. *The Underground Guide to Teenage Sexuality* (Basso, 1997), for example, written for adolescents, provides clear information on topics such as affectionate and sexual relationships, anatomical differences between men and women, physical and psychological (personality) transformation during adolescence, conception, pregnancy, and delivery, and all kinds of myths about sexuality. The book also provides information for parents. The *Life Horizons I and II* programme (Kempton, 1999) for adults and adolescents includes a series of slides on physiology and the sexual organs – photographs are useful for making information more concrete and avoiding misunderstandings. Details of the programme can be found at *www.stanfield.com*.

It is important to use the exact sexological terminology and its colloquial counterparts when discussing these various topics. The adolescent with AS is likely to know several of the scientific terms to describe sexual organs and behaviours (especially if he or she has a fondness for encyclopaedic information!), but it is preferable to use the more informal terms to allow him or her to associate more than one word with a given concept. Being too rigid could be quite harmful: colloquial terms must be accessible to individuals with AS so that they can interact equally with their peer group. This certainly does not mean that vulgar language should be used to talk about sexuality. The idea is to be open to colloquial language so as to avoid stigmatization or rejection by peers.

The Calgary Birth Control Association (2002) produced a detailed document on sexual health and education in a similar vein. Some of the key points, for example physical changes in puberty and hygiene, are presented below.

Physical changes in girls

In girls, puberty is marked by the menarche, the first menstruation, which indicates that the reproductive system has reached maturity. Physiological symptoms such as abdominal cramping, disturbances of the bowel, breast tenderness, and headaches can accompany the first period. These symptoms are temporary and can be alleviated by healthy eating habits and exercise. In some cases, medication (e.g. Anaprox, Midol, etc.) can be used to relieve discomfort. The physiological changes observed during puberty are due to the presence of sex hormones (oestrogen and progesterone). These trigger breast development, vaginal discharge (of a whitish colour), hair growth (on the pubis, armpits, legs, forearms, etc.), and, in some adolescents, pimples or acne. Muscle and bone mass increase and the hips widen.

A daily personal hygiene routine is recommended (see also p.24), since the surge in hormone levels causes a variety of bodily secretions (vaginal discharge, perspiration, etc.). Menstruation is a result of the shedding of a thin layer of cells of the endometrium (the lining of the uterus). The function of the endometrium is to receive the foetus. If conception doesn't occur, this lining and blood are shed through the vagina every month. Sanitary napkins are recommended and are easy to use. They should be changed every two to four hours or depending upon the menstrual flow. If the flow is light, the sanitary pad should be changed when it is full. Tampons can also be worn when the adolescent feels ready to insert an object into her vagina. Tampons should never be used at night, to avoid the risk of toxic shock; a sanitary pad should be worn instead. A demonstration is useful in teaching tampon use: show a tampon and explain where it should be placed. Models or drawings of the female genitals are appropriate for this (see Workshop 4). Family Planning Queensland (www.fpq.com.au) has developed a series of educational pamphlets, one of which is entitled "About periods" and shows how to use sanitary napkins. Vaginal douches or feminine deodorant sprays should be avoided as they increase the risk of developing vaginal irritation or an infection. Instead, a mild soap should be used to clean the genitals on a daily basis. It is normal for menstrual blood to give off an odour, which is why it is important to have good hygiene habits. Personal comfort and contact with others will be all the better for it!

The changes related to puberty must be addressed in a direct manner: information should be concrete, practical, and include images. The Family Planning Queensland brochures are very useful in this regard. If adolescents express apprehension or anxiety about menstruation they may find it useful to visit a doctor or a counsellor at the local community health centre. Having the information presented by a professional may well have a positive effect.

Young women with AS may react in different ways to breast development, on both a sexual and an interpersonal level. Given the visibility of this change, some young women will be thrilled with the transformation, a true sign of femininity. Having breasts can reassure the young woman of her gender identity (the sense of being a female) and of her sexual difference. Some young women value all aspects of femininity (clothing, make-up, hair, accessories, etc.). However, some are apprehensive about puberty and the bodily changes that accompany it. In that case, breast development can cause anxiety and thereby contribute to the emergence of inappropriate behaviours.

> Annie, a 13-year-old, flatly refused to wear her first bra, since this confirmed that she had breasts. In her class, boys made fun of girls with breasts. She therefore chose to wear loose clothing and tried to look like a boy in order to avoid their teasing. A couple of days later she leafed through a magazine containing pictures of movie stars wearing bathing suits. These images were quite confusing for her in that she noticed that the women in bathing suits had rather large breasts. She became anxious and started to examine her breasts every morning for fear that she would awake to a bad surprise: sudden big breasts. At school she lifted up her sweater to prove to classmates that she didn't wear a bra. All of the events became interwoven to such an extent that Annie expressed several signs of anxiety.
>
> A two-step intervention was organized in order to address the situation. First, Annie was provided with general information on puberty, including:
>
> - changes that take place during adolescence (hormones, gradual transformation of the body, pubic and underarm hair, bodily secretions, etc.)
> - changes she noticed that she found positive (she liked being taller than her sister, having muscles, and using antiperspirant).
>
> Second, Annie was presented with a series of pictures of young women wearing bras. These were clipped from a variety of fashion magazines and clothing catalogues. The goal was to show her the differences in breast size of young women and to explain that, in general, breast size is proportional to body size. That is, a woman who has a "medium" body size will have medium-sized breasts. On a dress size chart, Annie was able to find her body size and the breast size that she might expect to have (Table 1.1).

The intervention was reinforced using images from magazines (fashion, lingerie) showing various models of bras and different breast sizes. The images of the movie stars were used to introduce to Annie the concept of breast implants. She grasped this notion and understood that she wouldn't suddenly wake up with an imposing chest.

Table 1.1 Women's bra and dress sizes

Bra size					
Can/USA/UK	32A, B, C	34A, B, C	36A, B, C	38A, B, C	40A, B, C
France	85	90	95	100	105
Europe	70	75	80	85	90
Dress size					
	XS	S	M	L	XL
Can/USA	4–6	6–8	8–10	10–14	14+
UK	6–8	8–10	10–14	14–16	16+
France	0	1	2	3	4
Europe	34–36	36–38	38–42	42–44	44+

Physical changes in boys

Boys also experience multiple signs of puberty. The testicles increase in size (with shape and size varying from one adolescent to the next) and sperm production begins. The penis lengthens and widens. The length of the flaccid (non-rigid) penis is not related to the size of the erect penis. The length of an erect penis varies between 2½ and 8 inches (6–20cm), which is completely normal; the average size is between 5 and 7 inches (12–18cm). Some adolescents are curious or fearful about the size of their penis, the ultimate symbol of masculinity. It may be important to provide adolescents with basic information about the penis and to show them several types (different shapes and sizes, lengths, skin colours) so that they understand that genitals vary in appearance. The examples shown in books on sexual education are often not sufficiently representative or explicit. *The Penis Book* (Cohen 1999) is entertaining and very useful to this end. The penis is presented in historical context, in works of art, and in a variety of illustrations. The Internet site *www.thepenisbook.com* can also be used as an interesting accompaniment to the book. Ejaculation (expulsion of seminal fluid from the urethral opening) and nocturnal emissions are common, and general information on these is also included in Cohen's book.

Puberty is accompanied by a rapid growth spurt which can lead to fatigue, increased appetite, and clumsiness. The voice can change or remain the same. As with girls, hair growth and bodily secretions increase, underscoring the importance of a good daily hygiene routine. Family Planning Queensland's (2001) fact sheet on puberty explains these changes and can serve as a good reminder for the daily hygiene routine.

Hygiene

Some adolescent boys and girls with AS have problems with hygiene. Neglecting this area can have consequences for both health (infection, irritation) and interpersonal relations (avoidance, rejection, and stigmatization). To prevent these difficulties, the steps that lead to a good daily hygiene routine can be presented in the form of a reminder checklist (Figure 1.1). The boxes are ticked off on a daily basis and this helps adolescents become more responsible for their own hygiene practice.

Steps to good hygiene	Monday		Tuesday		Wednesday		Thursday		Friday		Saturday		Sunday	
	A.M.	P.M.	A.M.	P.M.	A.M.	P.M.	A.M.	P.M.	A.M.	P.M.	A.M.	P.M.	A.M.	P.M.
Hair														
Body														
Face														
Teeth														
Clean clothing														
Menstruation (change sanitary pad every 2–4 hours)														

Figure 1.1 Checklist for daily hygiene routine

In some cases, it may be preferable to use mild and perfume-free products, especially if the adolescent's sense of smell is very sensitive. For others, perfumed and colourful products may be a source of pleasure and serve as a good reinforcement. Many young women enjoy using delicately scented bath and body products. It is important to try a variety of products if the adolescent refuses to bathe. If the teenager has allergies or sensitivities to commercial products, "natural" products are another option. Natural vegetable-based soaps and shampoos are more expensive but less harmful to sensitive skin. Companies such as the Body Shop offer a variety of colourful herbal and glycerine-based products (soaps, body lotions, antiperspirants) that adolescents enjoy.

Responsibility and decision making

Some adolescents with AS have difficulty accepting the changes related to puberty because these represent what they fear about growing up (becoming an adolescent, an adult). This fear can be linked to anxieties associated with the responsibilities or decision-making that accompany adolescence. Listing benefits associated with adolescence can be a useful way of countering fears and discussing the advantages of puberty. Examples could include a later bedtime, riding a scooter, or earning pocket money by doing light tasks around the neighbour-hood (newspaper delivery, mowing lawns, gardening, washing cars, etc.). These earnings can then be used to purchase items to add to a collection (e.g. old albums, butterflies, books on the solar system, etc.). Outings can also become more interesting: joining a local bowling league or book club at the library; entering a chess tournament or enrolling in a painting class, etc. Using the young person's own particular interests to motivate them and to foster autonomy is a key element. Interpersonal relationships and social skills also need to be developed as much as possible, as discussed in Chapter 3.

Contraception

With the arrival of puberty, the reproductive system reaches maturity. This is therefore the opportune time to look at different methods of contraception. Kempton (1993) proposes the following three steps:

1. Present basic notions of contraception and pregnancy.

2. Discuss different means of contraception.

3. Prepare for a visit to a GP or gynaecologist (examination of internal and external sexual organs).

Contraception offers protection against unwanted pregnancy. No method is 100% effective, but with appropriate use the methods below are up to 98% effective (Calgary Birth Control Association, 2002; *www.cbca.ab.ca*). Abstinence (refraining from sexual intercourse), the safest sexual behaviour, is not a method of birth control but a personal choice.

- *Oral contraceptives ("the Pill")* can be up to 98% effective if used correctly. Each pill contains synthetic hormones that prevent monthly ovulation. When the adolescent takes her pill every day, ova (eggs) are not released from the ovaries, rendering conception impossible. Regular use of the Pill also brings about changes in the uterine lining which prevent implantation of the ovum. As with all methods of contraception, there are several advantages and disadvantages to taking the Pill. This information can be obtained from pharmacists, GPs, family planning clinics, product information leaflets, or pharmaceutical companies' websites.

- *Depo-Provera injections* contain progestin, a synthetic version of the hormone progesterone (a female sex hormone). A GP gives the injection every three months. It acts in the same way as oral contraceptives. Details, advantages, and disadvantages should be discussed with a GP.

- *Condoms* prevent pregnancy in 85 to 88% of cases and, if used in conjunction with a spermicide that contains Nonoxynol-9, effectiveness increases to 95%. Condoms are effective, affordable, and appropriate for adolescents. Proper use of a condom is presented in Workshop 7 of the sexual education programme.

- *Other means of contraception* include female condoms, intrauterine devices (IUD), and Norplant implants. They are described on the Calgary Birth Control Association's (2002) website, in Durocher and Fortier's (1999) sexual education programme, in the Family Planning Queensland (2001) brochure entitled "Contraception choices", and in family planning clinic leaflets.

Several of these methods of contraception are simple and effective. Adolescents should be given the freedom to choose which method they prefer (based on cost, ease of use, suitability, and accessibility). Condoms and birth control pills are generally the two methods most popular with teens. If used appropriately, the combination of these two methods is effective both for birth control and the prevention of sexually transmitted diseases (STDs). It is important to make sure that adolescents fully understand the different steps involved in their use. A vast number of information brochures are available in health clinics, hospitals, and family planning organizations.

Medical and gynaecological examinations

Medical and gynaecological examinations can be quite stressful for young women with AS. They need to be informed about and prepared for their visit to the doctor. The purpose of the gynaecological examination is to ascertain that the internal organs (vagina, cervix, uterus) and external organs (vulva, outer and inner labia) are normal. This is of utmost importance in identifying potential health problems early and preventing them from becoming more serious.

It is important to teach adolescents to develop a responsible attitude towards sexuality. For this to happen, they must be given as much information as possible on sexual development. This also prevents misunderstandings and mis-interpretations of issues surrounding puberty. A gynaecological exam can be a practical way of achieving this. The health professional can explain the changes that accompany puberty (hormones, secondary sexual characteristics, STD and HIV prevention, reproduction, etc.). Care must be taken to choose someone/a doctor who is comfortable with and knowledgeable about discussing sexuality in this way. When you make the appointment, explain the situation and ask the health professional to have additional informational pamphlets and brochures to hand. Explain to the adolescent that this visit to a doctor will be an opportunity for her to ask questions. Birth control can also be addressed during this medical visit – effectiveness and method of use of the various means of contraception can thus be explained in an appropriate context.

If the young person refuses to go to a doctor, a sexual health counsellor or sexologist can provide the same information without conducting the medical examination. Ask the adolescent what she prefers and encourage her to follow through. She is more likely to accept the appointment knowing that she is seeing a specialist. This is especially true given that individuals with AS tend to appreciate and value the opinions and scientific knowledge of professionals. If the adolescent is strongly resistant, this routine examination can be carried out in the school infirmary. The familiar surroundings of school can help decrease the teenager's anxiety. It is important to remember that, although this kind of examination should be encouraged to help the young woman better understand her development, it should not become a major source of stress.

While the exam can be very positive, it is by no means obligatory: it is always possible to delay the appointment and wait for a time when the adolescent is more receptive. Rather than risk creating a negative association between the examination and sexuality, it is better to wait for a more opportune time to make the experience much more valuable. Of course, the situation is quite different if an infection or another health problem is present.

Social influences

Image

Adolescents are usually quite concerned about the image that they project. Fashion, trends, and peer groups play an important role. The typical behaviours associated with adolescence can be experienced quite differently in teens with AS. For example, the desire to be part of a group of friends is much less pronounced, and trends in clothing, music, attitude, language, and so on can have very little impact on them. Individuals with AS perceive and integrate social rules quite differently. Two reactions are commonly observed: the teen is either not influenced by the peer pressures, or else conforms to them quite literally. In the latter case, behaviour, attitudes, or fashion trends are exaggerated, as in the following case example:

> Jimmy is 16 years old and possesses characteristics of AS (e.g. communication difficulties, circumscribed interests, interpersonal difficulties, difficulty controlling emotions). At the beginning of the school year he notices a group of kids his age listening to hip-hop music, wearing black jackets with a fur collar and baseball caps worn backwards. One of them says "hi" to him and invites him to a party. Jimmy immediately asks his parents to buy him new clothes (like those worn by the group of kids), but they refuse, since he refused to change his old clothes (always the same pair of jeans and comfortable white t-shirt) the previous week. He throws a tantrum and

promises his parents that he will wear his new clothes for the whole school year, without fail. At the party, several kids comment on Jimmy's clothes (he doesn't have the same logo on his baseball cap as they do).

Jimmy hadn't stopped to think about what he really wanted to wear, but rather focused on what the group seemed to prefer. When choices are rigidly dictated by society, trends, or a peer group, individuals with AS risk getting trapped into making impulsive decisions which can lead to rejection, especially when their relationships are based solely on style or belonging to the "in" crowd.

Taste in clothing can be developed by giving young people with AS the chance to choose what they prefer. Take the example of Sophie, a 17-year-old who had always received nasty comments about her attire. Her preference was for vintage clothing in varying shades of brown. Having worn the same clothes for several years, she noticed that other girls her age had adopted a very different style. After looking through a stack of fashion magazines for adolescents, Sophie decided to change her hairstyle. She got her hair cut and streaked with shades of red. People in her peer group reacted very positively to the change (her parents, however, were less thrilled with the radical new image!) and she chose to buy an outfit (vest and jeans). When I next saw her at a coffee house for people with AS, I didn't recognize her and in fact thought that she was a new counsellor. The change was amazing! Several young women approached her to ask where she had gone shopping. These reactions had a very positive effect on Sophie, who began to feel more confident and comfortable with herself. Such changes need to be encouraged when they occur, especially when they are self-initiated.

Self-esteem

Adolescence is also the period when self-esteem develops, and at this time adolescents with AS need the opportunity to express their conflicting feelings, experiences, worries, and preoccupations, including those relating to their sexuality. Parents and professionals close to them need to welcome their "difference" and encourage them to develop their strengths and special capabilities. However, during this period adolescents are extremely sensitive to what others think of them, and while they need to develop an image of themselves that is positive and not "deficient", their interpersonal difficulties only increase their feelings of rejection, often on a daily basis, as in the following example:

Luke is 14 years old and has been struggling to finish high school. He has had poor academic results and has been failing French and maths for the past three years. He therefore finds himself with 12- and 13-year-old classmates with whom he shares few interests. He prefers to withdraw into his "own world" which consists of computer drawings and electronic parts. He is unhappy at school and feels as though he doesn't fit in.

> Luke feels trapped. He doesn't make any attempts to meet other students at school because he figures that it is pointless since he always goes back to the same class, with younger classmates, regardless of what he does. His distress turns to generalized aggression towards all the kids at school. He can't stand to watch little groups of friends walking around and doing things together. He feels rejected and abnormal.

Teenagers like to be with other kids their age. They are often quite critical of those younger than them and don't appreciate contact with those in the grades below them. In particular, adolescents with AS frequently prefer the company of adults with whom they feel they can have an intellectual exchange. They feel that younger children prefer to play rather than learn or explore new electronic gadgets.

Also, Attwood (2003b) has noted that individuals with AS have difficulty recognizing emotion on the human face. In fact, they interpret signs (gestures, words, looks) quite literally, which leads to much misunderstanding and an overly rigid understanding of social interactions, which also accounts for Luke's vulnerability to feeling rejected by other adolescents and being aggressive towards them as a result.

> Interventions with Luke focused on teaching him basic friendship skills (saying hello, initiating a conversation, showing interest towards others, sharing, etc.) and how to take the initiative. He gradually gained more confidence in himself and agreed to participate in a party organized by some children at school. He felt so good when he received the invitation that his aggression was transformed to joy.

Self-esteem develops through relationships with others, but before entering into a relationship with someone else, it is important that adolescents feel good about themselves. Interpersonal exchanges are desirable as they help adolescents learn about themselves and their way of being with others. They develop social skills and friendships, and their emotional needs are met.

In adolescents with AS, anxiety and shyness hinder social contacts, their experiences in social situations are limited, and consequently their self-esteem is low. Withdrawal, isolation, or flight into circumscribed interests make young Aspies susceptible to feelings of depression, and the more they are confronted with their difficulties and constant experience of relationship failures at school, work, or in clubs and societies, the more they will avoid interpersonal relationships as a defence mechanism. Ultimately, the fear of behaving wrongly or of making mistakes can lead to social phobia (Attwood, 2003b) and, over time, specific subjects of interest become the only area in which the adolescent feels understood, competent, or appropriate.

This is Peter!

Coping with emotions, social narratives, and cognitive-behavioural therapy adapted to individuals with AS (Attwood, 2003a) are useful interventions, and young people with AS should be encouraged to express their emotions. Disappointment, fears, sadness, and aggression need to be expressed to avoid being transformed into inappropriate behaviours.

Sexual behaviour

Adolescence is marked by a desire to explore and experiment with different sexual behaviours. Individual, family, and cultural differences also influence sexual development. Adolescents with AS are curious too, but according to Griffiths (1999) and Hingsburger (1993), four factors have an additional impact on their sexuality. These must be considered if we are to understand better the complex sexual development of young people with developmental disorders.

- *Lack of sociosexual knowledge* is the first of these factors. Sociosexual knowledge plateaus around the age of puberty (Griffiths, 1999); individuals with AS at that age have rarely attained the maturity of the average young adult. They do not have the same experiences as adolescents in the general population, whether at the level of gender identity (sense of belonging to one's gender) or at the level of interaction with other teenagers, especially those of the opposite sex. These youngsters are victims of social asexualization; their sexuality is not recognized, as if their condition has eliminated the possibility of sexuality. The hypersexualization observed in some adolescents can be viewed as a result of a lack of understanding of social conventions and the notion of consent. Their familial and social environment frequently denies that they have sexual needs. In addition, they have little social support – with whom can they share their experiences and feelings? Peers and parents can be uncomfortable with the subject of sexuality, which further contributes to isolation in social situations. On the one hand, these teenagers have sexual needs that they attempt to express, and on the other, their sexual behaviours are punished. This conflict often leads to inappropriate behaviours (Griffiths, Quinsey and Hingsburger, 1989). Adolescents with AS score lower on a sexual knowledge questionnaire (Durocher and Fortier, 1999) than adolescents in the general population (Hénault, Forget and Giroux, 2003). Some have full knowledge of very specific subjects (anatomy, transsexualism, hormones, etc.), but the general concepts surrounding sexuality are often misunderstood.

- *Sexual segregation* is experienced by many individuals with AS, be it in specialized establishments, support groups, or at school. Given the prevalence ratio of four or five men to one woman (which can increase to 10:1 in clinical settings; Attwood, 2003b), the opportunities for interacting with members of the opposite sex who also have AS remain quite limited. Adolescents and adults alike are confronted with this reality and the lack of female partners available. Homosexual and masturbatory behaviours can therefore result from unsatisfying or limited contact with members of the opposite sex. Griffiths (1999) stated that if sexual segregation were replaced by integration, these behaviours would change and resemble those observed in the general population. Social activities and contact need to be encouraged. The greater one's social network, the better the chance of meeting someone with whom one has interests in common.

- *Inconsistencies* in the policies of various establishments (e.g. schools, offices, etc.), in the application of such policies by staff, and in the formal and informal rules surrounding sexuality are confusing for individuals with AS. If no precise rules exist, who determines what behaviours are acceptable? AS individuals are frequently bombarded with inconsistent messages and rules that are not adhered to consistently by everyone, and punitive interventions often decrease the likelihood of acquiring responsible behaviour. Teams who work with adolescents should create an open atmosphere around the subject of sexuality by providing sexual education, preventing sexual abuse, and recognizing the possibility of sexual contacts (Griffiths, 1999). It is of vital importance to educate staff, counsellors, youth workers, and parents who may otherwise impart incorrect information about sexuality (Hingsburger, 1993).

- *Intimacy* refers to the opportunity to be alone with a friendly, romantic or sexual partner, but such occasions are rare for adolescents with AS (Griffiths, 1999). Adolescence can be a difficult time due to hormonal changes, the desire for independence, and the marked need to explore. The reality of this must also be considered for teens with AS, since they are also changing on these levels. Intimate moments are not necessarily limited to sexual contact: they also make it possible for teens to broaden their repertoire of interpersonal experiences. The goal is to provide them with time and opportunities to develop intimate relationships with others. For some, intimacy is not felt to be necessary or important and is replaced by attempts for physical closeness which are frequently frustrating for the partner. In other cases, sexuality becomes an obsession and a fixed behavioural routine lacking in diversity and intimacy (Aston, 2001).

Studies of sexual behaviours

Few studies have examined the sexual behaviour of individuals with AS. Hellemans and Deboutte (2002) cite Haracopos and Pedersen (1992) and Hellemans (2001), who state that individuals with high functioning autism have a very real need to meet a partner and experience interpersonal relationships. In addition, the majority show a marked interest in sexual intimacy. That social difficulties interfere with this desire for intimacy leads to frustration for these individuals and their partners. Despite the fact that people with AS often have less sexual experience than those in the general population (Hénault *et al.*, 2003), some sexual behaviours are quite frequent.

Between 63% and 97% of autistic individuals masturbate (De Myer, 1979; Haracopos and Pedersen, 1999; Kempton, 1993). One study, conducted with 100 parents of autistic adolescents, found that 60% of the teens displayed sexual behaviours and 35% displayed inappropriate sexual behaviours (Gray, Ruble and Dalrymple, 1996). Ousley and Mesibov (1991) studied 21 autistic individuals with no intellectual disability and noted that men showed more sexual interest than women. Difficulty with social rules, interpreting emotions, explicit language, and their lack of sexual experience were all major stumbling blocks for the expression of this interest. Men tended to masturbate but were still quite frustrated because their desire remained. Masturbation is also the most frequent sexual behaviour for individuals with AS who are not looking for interpersonal physical or sexual contact (Aston, 2001).

Another study conducted with 89 autistic adults at various levels of development found that 65% practised masturbation (Van Bourgondien, Reichle and Palmer, 1997). These results are supported by those of Haracopos and Pedersen (1999) who, similarly, found a 67% rate of masturbation in a sample of 81 individuals with various levels of severity of autism.

Masturbation

Masturbation is the most common sexual behaviour reported by adolescents with AS. Discovering one's own body and the accompanying pleasant sensations is quite widespread. In and of itself, self-stimulation is not a problem, especially if expressed within acceptable contexts. However, behavioural problems related to masturbation are often observed in individuals with AS: Hellemans and Deboutte (2002) found that public masturbation is the most frequent inappropriate behaviour in autistic populations.

Masturbation can become a sexual compulsion or a source of distraction (just like any other activity). Some individuals achieve such pleasure that they constantly seek to reproduce it in order to distract themselves. They tend to engage in this behaviour when their level of general stimulation is not high enough (at school, work, or during free time).

In general, teens masturbate one to five times per day. Several factors contribute to the frequency of self-stimulation: the high levels of sex hormones (testosterone and oestrogen) characteristic of adolescence cause an increase in sexual desire, and orgasm and the physical pleasure that accompanies masturbation serve as powerful reinforcers.

Masturbation is usually discovered quite naturally, but information, support, and intervention may be needed. Shyness, shame, or guilt sometimes interferes, and the messages about masturbation can be contradictory – portraying it as dirty and unhealthy on the one hand, and a natural and desirable way of discovering one's body on the other.

According to Hingsburger (1995a), a number of behaviours or attitudes lead to problematic masturbation, including:

- the individual masturbates incessantly

- masturbation that does not end with ejaculation

- the individual masturbates but believes that it is bad, dirty, immoral, dangerous, disgusting, etc.

- injury occurs from masturbation (due to overly intense stimulation)

- masturbation in public

- the individual is afraid of masturbation.

Adolescents or adults with AS may display these behaviours or have difficulty forming their own opinion about the subject. Blum and Blum (1981) (cited in Hingsburger, 1995a) suggest five learning objectives with respect to masturbation:

- Learning that masturbation is a normal and healthy behaviour.

- Learning the appropriate time and place in which to engage in the behaviour (private versus public places).

- Debunking myths and their effects.

- Introducing the notion that sexual fantasies can accompany masturbation.

- Learning what kind of stimulation leads to pleasure.

This kind of education allows individuals with AS to express their emotions and any difficulties that they may have with self-stimulation.

Providing clear and concrete information is critical. The *Hand Made Love* guide and video (Hingsburger, 1995a) are interesting pedagogical tools for males, presenting sinformation on sexual health, emotions, fears, and myths surrounding masturbation. The goals of the video are to:

- provide pertinent information on male sexuality (on a behavioural level)

- create a welcoming and respectful atmosphere for the expression of sexuality

- provide information on physiology

- emphasize the private nature of masturbation.

You can also distribute Box 1.1, "Instructions for male masturbation".

Some adolescents are unable to ejaculate during masturbation, and lack of stimulation, tactile hyper- or hyposensitivity, or lack of skill can interfere with climax. Sexual excitation can reach the plateau phase and return to baseline without having reached orgasm (for a representation of the sexual response cycle see Workshop 4).

If ejaculation doesn't occur, testicular pain (epididimitis, or inflammation of the vas deferens, the canal that leads away from the epididimis), anxiety, or frustration can sometimes be experienced. Sometimes objects used can harm the genitals. Watching an educational video can sometimes help individuals learn the kinds of techniques that lead to successful stimulation, but any such educational activity should emphasize self-respect and privacy. It is always possible to stop the video if individuals are uncomfortable. The young man in the *Hand Made Love* video explains all the important steps (being alone in a private place, taking the necessary time, rhythm, touch, bodily sensations). This educational tool is not at all exhibitionistic and was developed especially for male adolescents and adults with AS.

Finger Tips (Hingsburger and Haar, 2000) is an educational guide and accompanying video for women. Its objectives are the same as those of *Hand Made Love* and the visual material is very useful for demystifying female masturbation. You can also distribute Box 1.2, "Instructions for female masturbation". Female self-stimulation is rarely addressed due to the many taboos that surround it. Prejudice about unbridled sexuality, lack of self-control, and nymphomania are sometimes raised. According to Masters and Johnson (1988, cited in Haracopos and Pedersen, 1999), 75% to 93% of women masturbate regularly. In young autistic women, the rates drop to 40% to 80%. However, the US National Information Center for Children and Youth with Disabilities recommends the discovery of one's body, pleasure, and sexual health:

> Masturbation can be a way of becoming more comfortable with and/or enjoying one's sexuality by getting to know and like one's body...masturbation only becomes a problem when it is practiced in an inappropriate place or is accompanied by strong feelings of guilt or fears. (Sexuality Information and Education Council of the US, 1991, p.3)

Box 1.1: Instructions for male masturbation

Before you begin you must make sure that you are in a private place (such as your bedroom or the bathroom), the door is locked, and you are alone. Masturbation (caressing your penis) is a *normal* behaviour that is not dangerous. Most adolescents masturbate. This allows you to discover your body and to experience pleasure.

The following steps will help you to masturbate successfully:

1. Caress your penis with your hand moving from top to bottom (up-and-down motion).

2. If you feel too much friction, you can use a lubricant that will allow your hand to slide on your penis (K-Y Jelly or another water-based lubricant; *never* use a petroleum jelly such as Vaseline).

3. Continue stroking your penis for five to seven minutes or a bit longer – however long you feel like it.

4. You will increasingly feel more sensations until a white liquid is expelled from the urethral opening in your penis. This liquid is semen (sperm) – this is normal, and it means that you have finished masturbating.

5. Use a tissue (e.g. Kleenex) or a wet towel to wipe your penis.

You may not always ejaculate (expel white liquid from your penis) – this is also quite normal.

✓

Box 1.2: Instructions for female masturbation

Before you begin you must make sure that you are in a private place (such as your bedroom or the bathroom), the door is locked, and you are alone. Masturbation (caressing your vulva) is a *normal* behaviour that is not dangerous. Most adolescents masturbate. This allows you to discover your body and to experience pleasure.

The following steps will help you to masturbate successfully:

1. Caress your vulva and your clitoris with your fingers (or with a blanket or a pillow) using delicate movements.

2. If you feel too much friction, you can use a lubricant that will allow your fingers to slide easily on your vulva and clitoris (K-Y Jelly or another water-based lubricant; *never* use a petroleum jelly such as Vaseline).

3. Continue caressing your vulva until you are satisfied with the pleasure that you feel.

4. You may feel intense pleasure for a short time – this is an orgasm. Some women have them, others don't. Orgasm doesn't take place every time you masturbate.

5. When you are finished, use a tissue (e.g. Kleenex) or a wet towel to wipe your vulva.

Betty Dodson's *Sex for One: The Joy of Selfloving* (1996) is another useful tool by which to discuss female masturbation from a perspective of intimacy, self-discovery, and pleasure. In 1974, Dodson also published *Liberating Masturbation*, which contains drawings of the female genitals and poetry. Both books discuss women's body image and are wonderful complements to the video.

Other sexual behaviours

Van Bourgondien and colleagues (1997) noted a variety of sexual activities practised by autistic individuals, including deep kissing, caressing, and genital contact. They found that 34% of those questioned had attempted these various sexual behaviours with a partner. Konstantareas and Lunsky (1997) conducted a similar study with 15 autistic adolescents and adults of various levels and found that 26% of their sample had experienced sexual relations whereas 46% had tried a variety of other sexual behaviours and deep kissing. Between 40% and 80% of teenagers in the general population practise sexual behaviours (Masters and Johnson, 1988, cited in Haracopos and Pedersen, 1999). These four studies report that between 26% and 67% of autistic individuals express sexual behaviours. These findings confirm that this population has an active sex life.

A series of six studies carried out by Hellemans and Deboutte (2002) with individuals on the autism spectrum found that the frequency of sexual behaviour in females was generally lower than that in males, owing to taboos, society's preconceived notions, sexual segregation, and lack of opportunity. Although results varied considerably between the six studies, they did suggest that most autistic women had given or received caresses, and up to two-thirds of them had kissed a partner. Sexual caresses were practised by up to nearly half of autistic women, but fewer than one-fifth of them had had sexual intercourse once or more. The studies also found that most men had experienced caressing or kissing, and nearly two-fifths of men had given or received sexual touch. Although these results are not specific to individuals with AS, they do paint a general picture of sexuality in autism. A sexual profile of individuals with AS determined on the basis of the sexual preferences, experiences, fantasies, and body image of 28 adults with AS can be found in the Appendix.

In conclusion, young people with AS begin the process of sexual maturation from the very first signs of puberty. From that moment on, physiological changes, self-esteem, and social interactions take on a whole new meaning. The desire to explore and experiment with sexuality is normal, but can lead to certain difficulties. Communication and openness about sexuality are your best allies. A variety of tools and interventions are proposed in the following chapters and additional resources are provided.

Chapter 2

Inappropriate sexual behaviours: Comprehension and intervention

Individuals with AS may have difficulty judging the appropriateness of expressing a sexual behaviour in a given context. A variety of other factors may also contribute to the development and persistence of inappropriate sexual behaviours. This chapter examines these factors and provides information on behaviours such as a specific interest in sexuality, sexual obsessions and compulsions, excessive self-stimulation, sexual aggression and criminal acts.

Precipitating and maintaining factors

The daily lives of people with AS are filled with misunderstanding, and these can result in a variety of inappropriate behaviours. The occurrence of such behaviours could be caused by a variety of factors, such as the setting, environment, and the individuals involved, and it is difficult to predict how a given context will influence a chain of events.

Flexibility and the ability to modify one's actions, usually make it possible to adjust one's behaviour to a given situation, but people with AS have difficulty judging appropriateness, as in the following examples:

> An adult with AS attended a street fair where musicians and artists performed. He yelled "That singer corresponds exactly to my fantasies!". He didn't consider that this comment, which might have been acceptable in a private conversation with a friend, was inappropriate in a public context.

> One woman with AS refused to answer her doctor's questions about her lifestyle and sexuality because she felt that they were indiscreet. She said, "I don't talk about those things with men that I barely know."

Some couples find that intimate contexts can also lead to disagreements because intimacy and romance can be experienced quite differently by each partner. While a walk by a lake may be seen as romantic by a neurotypical (non-Asperger) individual, it may be viewed as an opportunity to study water quality, wildlife, and flora by the partner with AS, who happily explains the changes in ecosystem. The moment loses its "romantic" value for the neurotypical partner because of the ecology lecture. The notion of context is quite vague and problematic for many individuals with AS, who lack the ability to decode the relevant elements that would inform them about the intimate context: the time, romantic location or other feature of the outing, needs of their partner, etc.

In other cases, inappropriate behaviours are triggered by specific factors. Individuals with AS don't intentionally act to provoke or shock, but changes in routine, for example, can be destabilizing to the point of provoking a tantrum. Environmental factors can act as stressors (e.g. noise, crowds, excessive demands, not understanding a situation, etc.) and cause withdrawal or aggressive behaviours.

Sexual frustrations are also sometimes expressed as inappropriate and aggressive behaviours. Several authors (Deslauriers, 1978; Gillberg, 1984; Hellemans and Deboutte, 2002; Kempton, 1993; Mesibov, 1989; Mortlock, 1989, all cited in Roy, 1996) have commented on the sexual difficulties encountered by individuals with a developmental disorder or AS. These individuals have enough difficulty interpreting their own emotions, let alone those of others in complex interpersonal relationships. They try, but fail, to imitate social behaviours. They feel sexual impulses just like everyone else, but some individuals with AS don't feel any meaningful sexual sensations or else experience sensory hypersensitivity.

Hypersensitivity and hyposensitivity

Individuals with AS can experience hypo- or hypersensitivity in their sense of hearing, smell, touch, taste, or sight, or of movement, proprioception, and balance (Smith Myles *et al.*, 2000). One sense is often overdeveloped to compensate for any loss in another. "Hypersensitivity" can be defined as extreme sensitivity in one or several of the five senses (hearing, smell, touch, taste, and sight) which are so important in sexuality. In AS, auditory and tactile hypersensitivity are very common and can be associated with neurological disorders (Asperweb France, 2000). For example, background music, played at the lowest volume setting, can be experienced as shrill and loud. Similarly, a very light touch can provoke the same pain as that caused by a cutting object. Clearly, such over-sensitivity can hinder sexual relationships by causing discomfort and even pain. Avoiding contact can further increase isolation and symptoms of depression.

Tactile sensitivity is reflexogenic and can serve two functions: protection and/or discrimination (or differentiation). Differentiation takes place very early in development when young babies use their senses to explore the environment. The protective function (usually the case in AS), leads to tactile defensiveness. This explains why a light touch or contact with certain fabrics can cause pain. In contrast, pressure is often perceived as soothing (Aquilla, 2003).

Tactile hypersensitivity can cause vaginal penetration to be painful for some women with AS. This pain is comparable to that experienced by women with vulvar vestibulitis syndrome (VVS). Symptoms of VVS include a burning, stinging pain at the entrance of the vagina. The treatment for VVS consists, in part, of preventing irritation or infection by re-establishing the vaginal flora. Practical suggestions for reducing vaginal irritation are listed below.

- Use little detergent on underwear and avoid fabric softener.

- Wear white cotton underwear; avoid synthetic fabrics (such as Lycra, Spandex).

- Wear loose trousers (avoid tight-fitting trousers, jeans, or pantyhose that may put pressure on the vulva).

- Remove wet clothing rapidly (bathing suits, exercise clothing).

- Avoid using scented products (bubble bath, sanitary products, feminine deodorant sprays, vaginal douches).

- Use water and mild soap on the genital area (for example, Dove, Ivory, or glycerine-based soaps).

- If penetration is painful, the use of a water-based lubricant such as K-Y or Astroglide may be useful.

- Topical anaesthetics, such as Xylocaine or EMLA, applied to the vulva, may decrease sensation.

In contrast, "hyposensitivity" is defined as a weak sensory response to stimuli. In these cases, over-exposure to stimuli is required for individuals to fully feel them. According to Aquilla (2003), these reactions are due to the slow transfer of sensation between nerve endings in the skin and the brain. Hyposensitivity can increase the probability of inappropriate behaviours. For example, individuals with AS often resort to masturbation, which provides a great number of very intense genital caresses, in order to feel sexual pleasure. Masturbation can therefore be misinterpreted as a sexual obsession or compulsion when it is, in fact, the result of a sensory phenomenon.

Smith Myles *et al.* (2000) have commented on the impact of hyper- and hypo-sensitivity on interpersonal relationships and emotions. They interpret these sensory reactions in a variety of ways and offer intervention strategies for each of the senses. Although they don't discuss sexuality, their book is a useful and practical resource for individuals with AS.

Worksheet 5.4 in the sexual education programme (Workshop 5) helps establish the sensory profile of individuals with AS. Sensory responses to visual, auditory, cutaneous, gustatory, and olfactory stimuli can be obtained in the guise of a game. The profile helps determine the impact of sensory responses on sexual behaviour.

Medication

The individual's medical history is an important source of information about inappropriate sexual conduct. Infections of the urogenital tract can cause tingling and inflammation of the pelvic region. A person with AS who constantly touches his or her genitals could be responding to itching sensations. Cutaneous relief should therefore not be confused with sexual stimulation (Griffiths, 1999). Organic factors appear to be involved in 25% of behavioural problems (Laxer and Tréhin, 2001).

Medication can also affect sexual function or cause side effects, for example, the drug Mellaril is frequently prescribed as a tranquillizer and an anti-psychotic, but erectile dysfunction and retrograde ejaculation (semen in the bladder) are common side effects of its use (Alarie and Villeneuve, 1992). Individuals with AS frequently use more than one kind of medication, and combinations of drugs can have synergistic or problematic effects. Unfortunately, many medications are prescribed for patients with AS without anyone explaining the sexual side effects. The Internet site Virtual Hospital (*www.vh.org*) provides descriptions of diseases, infections, and side effects of a variety of medications. Such sites make it possible to obtain medical information quickly and free of charge.

Table 2.1 (p.42) shows the side effects of selected medications, listed in order of most to least frequent. Side effects are not the same for everyone since they largely depend on the individual's metabolism, and each individual reacts differently to medication. Higher doses lead to a greater risk of developing side effects. Side effects are not necessarily immediate or automatic; they can appear gradually after several weeks of taking a medication. It is important always to consult a physician or psychiatrist if a secondary sexual dysfunction occurs. There are two possible solutions: decreasing the dose or changing medication by staying in the same family of drugs. The therapeutic effects can be more important than the undesirable side effects.

Medication should *never be discontinued* and a dose should *never be modified* without first consulting a physician.

Some side effects are directly related to sexual functioning whereas others are linked to social functioning. Uncontrollable tics or dyskinetic movements, for example, increase the social isolation of people with AS.

Table 2.1 Side effects of medication on sexuality and sociability

Antidepressants

Luvox, Paxil, Effexor, Zoloft, SSRIs (selective serotonin reuptake inhibitors)
- decreased libido (sexual desire)
- erectile dysfunction (loss of penile rigidity)
- delayed ejaculation (only with Luvox if dose exceeds 150 mg per day)

Paxil *only*
- contraindicated for young people under 18 years of age due to increased suicide risk (Health Canada and GlaxosmithKline Inc., Government of Canada, 2003)

Antipsychotics (neuroleptics)

Mellaril, Serequel, Serzone
Mellaril *only*
- decreased libido
- erectile dysfunction (in 44% of cases)
- painful ejaculation or retrograde ejaculation (ejaculation into the bladder)

Risperdal
- erectile dysfunction
- difficulties with ejaculation/orgasm
- agitation/anxiety
- can cause dyskinetic and involuntary movements (with long-term use, depending on dosage, and if combined with another antipsychotic)
- can cause insomnia

Zyprexa
- symptoms of Alzheimer's disease may occur

Anxiolitics (anti-anxiety medications)

Buspar *only*
- increase or decrease in libido

Buspar, Rivotril
- drowsiness (in 50% of cases)
- behaviour disorders (in 25% of cases)

Benzodiazepines: e.g. Ativan, used to treat anxiety, nervousness, or tension (max. effect 60–90 minutes after medication is taken)
- drowsiness

For Attention Deficit Disorder with/without hyperactivity

Ritalin
- can increase pre-existing tics

Sources: Health Canada and GlaxoSmithKline Inc., Government of Canada, 2003; University of Iowa, 2003; Canadian Pharmaceutical Association (*www.autisme.qc.ca*), 1994; Alarie and Villeneuve, 1992; Paradis and Lafond, 1990.

Behavioural history

Inappropriate sexual conduct, paraphilias, deviant behaviours, aggression, excessive self-stimulation, and sexual compulsions are also found in individuals with AS. Griffiths, Quinsey and Hingsburger (1989) propose a variety of models to explain these sexual behaviours.

The behavioural history can contribute to the development of inappropriate sexual conduct. Griffiths (1999) reported the case of a young man with a developmental disorder who was punished each time he attempted to establish contact with a woman, even though the attempts were appropriate. He then forced a sexual contact on an unconsenting woman. He thought that there would be a lesser chance of being reprimanded if the gesture was quick. The gesture takes on a new meaning if we understand the reason for the behaviour. According to this man, his strategy was appropriate given the circumstances in which the behaviour was expressed.

Inappropriate behaviour sometimes seems to be the only course of action for an individual whose urges have constantly been repressed by society. The forbidden becomes attractive and problematic behaviours emerge (Griffiths, 1999; Hingsburger, 1993).

Modelling and imitation

Modelling and imitation can also lead to inappropriate conduct. Lack of discrimination on the part of individuals with AS can cause ritualistic behaviours to take place outside their normal context. Griffiths (1999) has provided examples of exhibitionism in individuals with pervasive developmental disorders (PDDs). In one case, a young woman left the door open when she went to the bathroom at school and put her clothes back on in the hallway on the way back to class. What could explain this behaviour? According to Griffiths, it was important to conduct a functional analysis of this inappropriate behaviour in order to understand it within the context of her daily life. What emerged from the analysis was the fact that she could not make the distinction between what could be done in private as opposed to public settings. Such poor interpretation of contextual cues by people with PDDs adds to their vulnerability (National Information Center for Children and Youth with Disabilities, 1992). The notion of "private" versus "public" is frequently misunderstood by people with AS. Gray and colleagues (1996) found that some individuals had never learned that personal hygiene is a private behaviour. They explained this phenomenon with the fact that people with AS are often used to having these needs attended to by others and therefore cannot differentiate between when and where they can and cannot expose themselves.

The behavioural repertoire of individuals with AS often consists of rituals and routines that make the person feel safe but that may become problematic in social situations. Interpersonal relationships are further complicated by poorly developed social skills. Individuals with AS tend to imitate the behaviour of their peers without necessarily understanding the complexity of the behaviour. As a result, much behaviour can be reproduced out of context. For example, a male with AS might, upon noticing a couple kissing on the street, kiss the first girl that he sees. He might also reproduce inappropriate behaviours that he has been subject to in the past. Some parents worry about their child's affectionate behaviour. One mother told me that her son had the habit of kissing blonde women on the cheek. This behaviour can be acceptable for a six-year-old child, but not for an adolescent. In order to discourage this behaviour, his mother limited his contact with blonde women to those he knew (e.g. his aunt and cousin). Since he had difficulty changing the behaviour, his mother rewarded him (with ice cream, computer time, or gifts for his toy car collection) each time he respected the rule of not kissing blonde women. Affectionate behaviour in childhood should have clear boundaries so that individuals with AS don't show inappropriate behaviours in adulthood. The distinction between public, private, and intimate behaviours needs to be explained to them so that they can learn to act according to the rules governing social behaviour. Failure to do so will increase the likelihood of individuals with AS finding themselves in uncomfortable or abusive situations or display sexual behaviours that are inappropriate in the context.

Partner selection

Individuals with AS are quite limited with respect to partner selection, especially since the 4:1 male to female ratio of AS makes it unlikely that they will find a partner who also has AS. In addition, many are isolated and have few friends. Communication difficulties, fear of rejection, and interpersonal anxiety also limit their social network. They sometimes develop romantic feelings towards counsellors or youth workers whom they see on a regular basis. This confusion seems quite normal given that these are the people who regularly care for them (Griffiths, 1999). Intimacy and attachment are natural by-products of this special relationship. It is therefore important for professionals and parents to encourage them to develop relationships with other people in order to broaden their circle of acquaintances. They can meet new people at dances, hobby-related activities, chess clubs, or collectors' conventions (for example). Despite their general resistance to new activities, it is to their benefit to meet a variety of people in the community and in clubs or other organizations. The goal is to break the pattern of isolation, develop friendships, and meet interesting new people and possibly a partner.

Imagination

During adolescence, their imagination can bombard young people with AS with all kinds of images and scenarios. They may therefore claim to be in love with an assortment of movie stars, singers, or media personalities. Such imaginary relationships allow them to express their feelings freely, without fear of rejection. Fantasies are orchestrated at their whim without the need to resort to the communication and social skills that are such a vital part of interpersonal relationships. Girls with AS often have imaginary friends (Attwood, 1998a). However, when the individual's fantasy life interferes with establishing relationships with people, feelings of failure and loneliness can ensue and increase depressive moods. An increased feeling of self-worth and an enriched imaginary life can be gained by developing real friendships.

Frustrations

Frustration is frequently expressed as inappropriate or aggressive behaviour. Individuals with AS regularly fail to understand requests made of them, and they may also have difficulty detecting or expressing their own internal changes (hormonal variations, emotional conflicts, changing moods, etc.). Such situations are rife with confusion and frustrations which may cause inappropriate behaviours. Impulsive actions may be the only means of releasing internal tensions. A functional analysis of aggressive or impulsive behaviours observes what took place prior to, during, and after the occurrence of these behaviours. This kind of descriptive analysis helps create an understanding of the purpose of behaviour by providing clues about what caused it. Aggressive behaviours can often be viewed as "symptoms" of frustration. Consider the following example:

> Morgan, a 20-year-old, desperately wanted to meet some boys at school. She tried approaching them, talking to them, invited some out on dates, but nothing seemed to work. One lunch time, she saw some young women talking to a group of guys. The next day, without any regard to context, she imitated the women's gestures and used the same words as they had to approach a group of guys. Since they were talking about something else, the young men told her to stop bothering them and go back to class. Morgan was disappointed and frustrated, and she threatened to beat up the young women and to make them pay for the rejection she had experienced.

This kind of need for revenge is dangerous insofar as innocent bystanders, who have had nothing to do with the individual with AS, could be at the receiving end of harsh words and gestures. Individuals with AS need to be made aware of the consequences of their words or actions. Complaints may be lodged against them and lead to complications. Their frustrations, expressed as aggressive or inappropriate behaviours, can also turn against themselves. Self-mutilation can take on several forms, such as hitting, cutting, and intentionally hurting oneself. Such behaviours can emerge during moments of high anxiety and rejection (Stoddart, 2003). When directed towards others, inappropriate behaviours take the form of aggression, sexual touching, harassment, provocation, or intimidation. To date, the prevalence of such behaviours in autism or AS has not been reported. However, some authors (De Myer, 1979; Gillberg, 1983; Hénault, Forget and Giroux, 2003; Wing, 1975 in Hellemans and Deboutte, 2002; Hellemans, 1996) report cases where public masturbation, inappropriate touch, sexual assault, and physical violence have taken place.

Interpreting emotions

Another precipitating factor is difficulty in interpreting emotions. Individuals with AS have great difficulty decoding emotions, both their own and those of others. Their understanding is usually limited to basic emotions such as joy, anger, or sadness. They need to explore the complete continuum of emotions in order to learn to express what they feel, since sexuality is associated with emotions that far surpass two or three basic emotions.

Understanding the subtlety of these many emotions enriches relations with others. During a conversation with a man in her activities group, a woman with AS could detect that he was experiencing joy because she could see he was smiling. In fact, the man had to explain to her that he was much more than happy: he fancied her. According to him, this was noticeable by the look in his eyes and his general attitude toward her. Learning about and decoding emotions is an important part of sexuality. The ability to express emotions and to interpret those of others reduces the frustration and impulsive reactions of individuals with AS.

Individuals with AS often feel their emotions physically (trembling, heart beats, sweating, etc.), and emotional cues (attachment, loneliness, etc.) are often difficult to interpret. Decoding others' emotions based on facial expression can be a great puzzle for some, and the subtleties of nonverbal language escape them, all of which increases the potential for misunderstandings. Approximately 30% of communication is verbal, whereas 70% is nonverbal; this partly accounts for the difficulties experienced by individuals with AS. In some cases, people with AS will use their imagination as a way to express emotions in the form of imaginary play, drawings, scenarios, or other seemingly bizarre acts. Due to their restricted emotional repertoire, their emotions frequently manifest themselves in an extreme manner; for example, sadness can be expressed as anger or aggression. Learning a broader range of emotions enhances expression and decreases intensity. The following two examples illustrate difficulties around the expression of emotion.

> Julian had AS, was 45 years old, and had been in a relationship with Marie for almost four years. His ex-girlfriend obtained custody of their daughter, which made him quite sad. During their first fight, Marie accused Julian of not expressing his feelings clearly. Since it was difficult for him to recognize

the physical and emotional cues associated with sadness, he tended to yell and get carried away rapidly. Simple misunderstandings ended in tantrums. Julian did not know any other way to express his feelings. Marie started to believe that he was always angry, until Julian finally realized that he was experiencing sadness, rather than frustration, over the separation and loss of his daughter whom he missed very much.

David, a 14-year-old, had recently been diagnosed with AS. He attended a special education class at his high school. He always behaved and expressed his emotions impulsively. Following a difficult break-up, he wrote a letter in which he explained, in detail, how he would physically harm all the girls at school. He left the letter on his desk, and his teacher found it. The gory details alarmed his teacher and she contacted his parents. When he was asked why he wanted to get rid of the girls at school, he responded, "Because I'm sad and lonely. Girls won't bother me as much if they aren't around."

Notwithstanding David's dramatic reactions, it is important to explore the emotions behind someone's behaviour before jumping to conclusions. The activities in the sexual education programme described in Part 2 (Workshops 3, 6 and 12) help individuals learn to decode physical and emotional cues and to broaden their emotional repertoire.

Interpersonal relationships

Interaction in human relationships takes place on so many different levels (emotional, nonverbal, verbal, cognitive, etc.) that it becomes quite complex, and the complexities of interpersonal relationships are often misunderstood. Individuals with AS have difficulty decoding all of the messages that are conveyed during a conversation or interaction involving several people: words and phrases with double meanings are confusing and leave them perplexed, and nonverbal language (which acts as a form of parallel communication) is also difficult to grasp. A simple conversation can therefore turn into a nightmare. Sexuality is filled with subtleties, little gestures, and intentions that must be decoded on yet another level. Individuals with AS have reported that they experience this much as they would someone speaking a foreign language: "It's like learning a new language each time." Some people will manage to find a reference point (key words, precise gestures, tone of voice) to help them decode messages. Nonetheless, misunderstandings are very common.

One way of learning to expand the repertoire of human emotions is to explore the levels of communication that we use. Through vignettes and simple role play, individuals can explore the different messages to be found in a given phrase. In the example "I like you, would you like to go out tonight?", the first interpretation is an invitation to go out (factual level); the second is the interest directed at me (emotional level); the third is related to the other's intention (interpersonal level); and the fourth is the nonverbal language (parallel communication found in gestures, smile, tone of voice, proximity, etc.) used. Using simple examples, all of these meanings can be explored in this way. Increasingly complex situations (in terms of message and number of interactions involved) can be presented. These activities should be conducted in a safe environment and emphasis is placed on the desire to interact with someone and not on performance. The greater the sense of competency experienced, the smaller the need to withdraw from personal relationships.

Promiscuity

Promiscuity is frequently observed in the behaviour of women with AS. Sexual promiscuity is defined as having sexual relations with several different partners, simultaneously or in succession, without considering the dangers of such behaviour (Département de Sexologie, 1996). Causal factors include lack of experience and boundaries, poor judgement, and deficits in theory of mind (capacity to imagine what the other is thinking). Some women with AS accept all sexual offers in an attempt to obtain affection and intimate contact, and some people take advantage of their naivety and vulnerability. Social networks, social skills, and sexual education can help women with AS learn how to deal with potential abusers. Role-playing helps to develop their judgement. Intervention strategies aimed at preventing sexual abuse are presented in Workshop 11.

Consent

"Consent" is defined as a mutual and willing agreement about any kind of sexual exchange. Sheehan (2002) examines the notion of consent in individuals with a PDD. She takes up McCarthy's (1993) definition which stipulates that an informed decision begins with knowledge of human sexual anatomy and physiology. Sexuality not only involves intercourse but various forms of pleasure from a variety of erogenous zones, and consent is not limited to sexual relations but to all forms of touch, including caresses to the genitals and other erogenous zones (mouth, breasts, buttocks, etc.). Sheehan (2002) lists eight factors which must be understood in order for an individual with a developmental disorder to be able to give consent.

- Sexuality is experienced with another person in a private place.

- Sexual contact with animals, children, individuals from the same family, or to obtain money, is inappropriate.

- Sexual relations can lead to pregnancy, which implies an emotional and economic commitment on the part of the parents.

- Methods of contraception, when used appropriately, decrease the risk of pregnancy.

- Methods of contraception are available from pharmacies and specialized clinics (family planning clinics).

- Unprotected sexual behaviours increase the risk of contracting a STD. Symptoms of STDs include irritation, discomfort, infection, and fever.

- People believe that sexuality should take place in a respectful and loving context.

- It is always possible to refuse to engage in sexual contact; it is a personal choice.

When notions of consent are poorly understood or not respected, individuals with AS can not only become victims of sexual assault or abuse, but may also perpetrate it. The deficits in their theory of mind increases their risk of committing an act of sexual assault since they may not take into account the other person's desires. If overly self-centred, individuals with AS don't consider the needs of others. This unfortunate situation is quite common in individuals with AS who have an impaired theory of mind and who don't understand the notion of consent.

> Zachary, an 11-year-old, was very curious about the female body. One day he was caught touching the genitals of one of the girls at his school. He had taken it upon himself to explore her body without warning her or obtaining her consent. She didn't have time to react because Zachary was quick and impulsive.

Interventions target understanding boundaries in social relationships. Narratives, cartoons, and social circles are among the tools used to explore the rules of intimate sexual behaviour. The person must understand very clearly that a series of questions must be answered before any intimate behaviour occurs. These include:

- What is my relationship to this person (stranger, friend, lover, authority figure)?

- What behaviour is involved (hand holding, peck on the cheek, touching a private body part, being caressed)?

- Does the other person have the same idea as me (does he or she wish to be intimate with me)?

- Is the behaviour appropriate for my age?

- Are there consequences to this behaviour?

- Are we in a private or public place?

- What is the context (school, park, home, special event)?

These questions can be integrated into narratives inspired by those of Carol Gray's (1994) Social Stories. Scenarios must be repeated several times to make sure that the person with AS understands. Repetition and multiple examples improve learning and subsequent generalization.

Sexual history

It is important to consider sexual history when discussing inappropriate sexual conduct. Sexual abuse is frequent in autistic and Asperger populations. The American Academy of Pediatics (1996) commissioned a study from the National Center on Child Abuse and Neglect who reported a mean of 36 cases of sexual abuse per 1000 children presenting with a developmental disorder. This rate is 1.7 times higher than that found in the general population. The limited social skills of individuals with AS result in a lack of experience and judgement, and their lack of sexual information and knowledge has a negative impact on notions of consent with respect to the sexual requests that they receive (Griffiths, 1999; Hingsburger, 1993; National Information Center for Children and Youth with Disabilities, 1992).

A history of abuse can also lead to the appearance of inappropriate sexual behaviours, since children or adolescents who have been abused may reproduce the behaviour of which they have been a victim. Thus adolescents who have experienced abuse in the form of sexual touching of the genitals may repeat this behaviour with another person because they fail to detect the intimate nature of the behaviour; they simply imitate it.

Understanding inappropriate sexual behaviours

When faced with several inappropriate behaviours, it is crucial to have a thorough understanding of the behaviours in order to devise an intervention strategy. Factors that influence inappropriate sexual conduct, as well as strategies for dealing with them, are shown in Box 2.1. Tréhin (2002) proposes the criteria shown in Box 2.2 for the global analysis of inappropriate behaviours in individuals with AS.

Restricted interests and sexual obsessions

Since individuals with AS have a propensity for repetitive and ritualistic activities, sexual behaviours may become their special circumscribed interest. It will be difficult to curb such an interest, especially if it is a source of pleasure and satisfaction. As long as their sexual interests do not cause any harm to the individual himself or to others, it is important to control but not prohibit access to

Box 2.1: Factors influencing inappropriate sexual behaviour

1. Comprehension

- *What conditions influence the behaviour?*
  Stress, anxiety, changes in routine, changes in personnel, reactions to an event, a learned behaviour that the individual tends to reproduce?

- *What is the reinforcement history?*
  In general, what are people's reactions, what are the consequences? What does the individual gain from the behaviour (attention, removal from an unpleasant situation)? Are there any secondary gains? Any reinforcing factors?

- *What purpose does the behaviour serve?*
  Attention, routine or ritual out of context, avoidance of a situation or an individual, challenging authority and rules, causing damage?

2. Causes

- Lack of comprehension regarding the environment (rules, expectations, interactions).

- Deficits in expression of needs (verbal, emotional).

- Organic factors – responsible for 25% of serious health problems (medication, illness).

- Physical pain (infection, irritation, discomfort).

- Associated psychological or psychiatric difficulties (comorbid factors such as personality disorders, schizophrenia, psychosis, generalized anxiety, depression, obsessive-compulsive disorder, post-traumatic stress disorder).

- Lack of activities/stimulation or over-stimulation.

3. Strategies

- Establish a communication system (in order to allow for verbal, nonverbal, and emotional expression).

- Explore the repertoire of emotions.

- Propose a behavioural alternative. Replace the problematic behaviour with behaviour which has the same value or function. Look at:
  - whether it is easy to learn and reproduce
  - its normative value (age, culture, valued by peers, etc.)
  - whether it can be carried out in another environment
  - whether it is incompatible with the inappropriate behaviour (ideally it should be).

Box 2.2: Possible causes of inappropriate behaviours in individuals with Asperger's Syndrome

Health/medical

- Don't know how to express pain.
- General poor health or non-localized problem (digestion, fatigue etc.).
- Epilepsy.
- Depressed state.

Sensory

- Over-stimulation or unpleasant sensations (sounds, lights, people, physical contact).

Communication

- Carrying out requests *literally*, not understanding others' irritation at result (literal understanding).
- Not understanding instructions and:
  - not knowing that they should *say* that they don't understand instructions
  - not knowing *how to say* that they don't understand instructions.
- Need help (don't know how to carry out or organize tasks):
  - don't know that they *have to ask* for help in order to obtain it
  - don't know *how to ask* for help in order to obtain it.
- Have to interrupt a task in progress in order to do what is requested.
- Poor understanding of or incomplete information (someone says that we are going to the grocery store but we stop at the post office on the way).
- Don't understand that others are joking.

Predictability/time

- Unfulfilled expectation (compared with prior experience).
- Changes to schedules without warning; assumptions based on information provided previously remained unfulfilled.
- Need for more time (slow, stressed by the demand).
- Difficulty understanding notions of time (understand "yes, *now*" instead of "yes, *this afternoon*").
- Failure of others to adhere strictly to schedules or agreed times (they were told that we would "leave at five o'clock", and at 5.01 p.m. we haven't left yet...).

Social

- Too much pressure, over-stimulation: having to pay attention to too many things and people.
- Don't think about the consequences of their actions or words.
- Don't know implicit rules of social interaction.
- Fear of failure.
- Difficulty controlling emotions (even positive ones).

Motivation/interests

- Effort isn't worth the results.
- Problem behaviour is reinforced by its consequence (positive/negative attention).
- Overwhelmed by obsessional interests.
- Inability to judge the relative importance of criticism (throw-away comments taken to heart may result in a permanent feeling of failure).

Adapted from Tréhin (2002) with permission

sexuality – to prohibit it will only serve to make it more appealing. It is important to remember that a surge in sexual interest during adolescence is normal in most young people and the mix of curiosity and excitement makes the discovery of sexuality very attractive. In order fully to understand their own sexual functioning, individuals with AS need to have sexual experiences.

Teenagers' need to explore must be respected – within reasonable limits – because it also signifies an interest in others. This developmental stage is perfectly normal and indeed desirable as it leads to socialization and the development of friendships or intimate relationships. Individuals with AS may or may not have this need for closeness, but if they do, they should not be prevented from experiencing it.

It is possible that sexuality can take on another dimension and become a veritable obsession, characterized by uncontrollable, disproportionate desires that may be accompanied by anxiety. This phenomenon is not present in all individuals with AS and few empirical data exist, but the author's clinical observations show that it is detectable in some individuals. In these cases sexuality becomes the only source of interest and stimulation to the detriment of all other activities. The obsession can take on a variety of forms: excessive use of pornographic materials (magazines, Internet, etc.), voyeurism, compulsive masturbation, seeking out sexual contact, excessive desire for closeness and repetitive fantasies, for example. If the obsessions are not satisfied (which is likely), the individual can become frustrated, isolated, and depressed.

When the obsession is accompanied by anxiety, the individual's universe revolves entirely around sexuality and has a detrimental effect on everything else, including work, other activities and their partner, if there is one. Take the example of an individual with AS who watches four hours of Internet pornography per day, masturbates at work during his breaks, constantly seeks sexual contact with women, and openly talks about the different sexual fantasies and scenarios that he would like to experience. Given that it is obviously impossible to live out one's sexuality at such a pace, a level of anxiety will be almost certainly experienced by this individual.

Carnes (1989) identified a variety of indicators that may be observed in an individual who has lost control over that obsessive interest in sexual behaviours:

- The individual has difficulty resisting potentially harmful sexual impulses, urges, or temptations (obsession).

- The individual feels an increase in tension and/or anxiety prior to acting out a sexual behaviour. The purpose of the act is to decrease this tension (compulsion).

- The individual experiences pleasure and tension release when the compulsive behaviour is performed, but can feel guilt and/or regret immediately afterwards.

- The individual has made repeated efforts to reduce, control, or stop the behaviour but these have been unsuccessful.

- Sexual activities occupy most of the individual's time and interfere with work and other obligations.

- The sexual behaviours occur regardless of physical (irritation, genital pain due to repetitive gestures) or financial (high cost of pornographic material) difficulties, or problems with a partner.

- The individual becomes irritable and distressed if the sexual behaviours cannot be performed.

These signs and symptoms must persist for at least one month and appear repeatedly over a long period of time.

Carnes (1989) also described three levels of sexual compulsions. The first is characterized by the obsession. Individuals mistakenly believe that they have control over the obsession and can, for example, resort to masturbation at the first sign of loneliness or frustration. Sexual relations are void of meaning, engaged in without joy or pleasure, and use of pornographic material or sex workers is excessive. The second level of sexual compulsion involves incurring a legal conviction – this becomes necessary when actions are perpetrated on a victim by the individual. For some, this risk factor adds to the excitement. This is true for exhibitionism, frotteurism, and obscene telephone calls. In the third and most serious level, the vulnerability of others is exploited, as in paedophilia, incest, and sexual assault. Carnes adds that an individual can engage in more than one level of compulsive behaviour in a given time period. Sexual compulsions can also transform to a compulsion for alcohol or drugs.

It is time to intervene when individuals experience a loss of control over their sexual compulsions. There are several intervention strategies that can be adapted to the profile of individuals with AS (Carnes, 1989, 1993; Coleman, 1991) and according to Carnes, group therapy should be the treatment of choice. Sexoholics Anonymous is based on the 12-step Alcoholic Anonymous (AA) model. Treatment goals include:

- admitting the problem

- modifying belief systems

- exploring new healthy and safe behaviours and strategies to avoid compulsions

- involving partners and family members

- breaking isolation.

Other intervention strategies target stress management, communication skills, self-esteem, and the exploration of intimacy and satisfactory sexual relations. The different treatments have varying success rates, but it is recommended to combine individual and group therapy (Swisher, 1995).

Of course each case is unique, but it is important to bear in mind that to punish the individual or to neglect tackling the situation will only cause any underlying anxiety to increase. Even if it is a difficult subject matter, individuals with AS should be encouraged to express what they are experiencing and explain how the situation occupies their mind. The impulse needs to be expressed to decrease the anxiety that it generates.

> Carl was 21 years old and had AS. He came to therapy for "sexual difficulties". When I inquired about what the difficulties were (it is important to be clear and explicit), he confided that he was totally obsessed by the idea of having sex. He had had sexual contacts with a 25-year-old woman a year ago, and hadn't been able to stop thinking about it since. In addition, he tried to meet women in every possible way. His desire was fuelled by a rich fantasy life and daily perusal of erotic magazines. He described himself as obsessed. His psychiatrist had prescribed medication to calm his obsessions but no change was apparent.
>
> Carl was encouraged to talk about his obsessions and to describe them in detail, with the aim of decreasing his anxiety. After four or five one-hour sessions, he described himself as less stressed because talking about the problem allowed him to defuse the situation rather than fuel his obsession.

Carl subsequently rejoined a group of young adults in their activities at a day centre. Since he was less anxious, his desire was less pressing (although still present). He behaved more appropriately with girls and was less direct in his demands. After a month he had made friends with a girl in the group whom he subsequently started dating. He reported that she too had the desire to have sexual relations with him. He explained how he had planned his first sexual encounter with his 20-year-old girlfriend: dinner in a restaurant, a movie, taking a hotel room and... That is exactly what happened! His only disappointment was that her body was quite different from those he had seen in magazines and he was so shocked by this that he couldn't help telling her. They talked about it and he decided to make do with the situation since there were several advantages to being with her (outings, activities, sexual contact).

If sexual behaviours in AS individuals take the form of an obsession, consider the following questions:

- What sexual behaviours are involved?

- How long has the obsession been present?

- Under what circumstances does the obsession express itself (time of day, preceding and following activities, individuals involved)?

- What purpose does the obsession serve?

- How does the individual behave when he or she talks about the obsession?

- What emotions accompany the repetitive behaviour(s): anxiety, anger, sadness, fear, joy, excitement?

The answers to these questions allow a functional analysis of the obsession to be carried out. Here are some possible interpretations:

- Sexuality is the only source of satisfaction, pleasure, excitement, or gratification for the individual.

- The sexual behaviour decreases the adolescent's anxiety (especially in situations where a lot is expected of him or her).

- Sexuality becomes a way to challenge authority or 'the forbidden'.

- Sexual activity is a way of behaving like an adult (the adolescent doesn't want to be considered a child).

- Sexual contact stimulates the sensory systems (tactile, visual, olfactory). An intervention strategy based on stimulation may be necessary if the individual with AS is hyposensitive. This would allow him or her to tolerate a minimum of stimulation.

- Sexuality is symptomatic of an underlying conflict (search for identity, frustration, peer rejection, romantic failures, or social isolation).

- Sexual behaviour is viewed as having the same value as any other behaviour. There are differences associated with sexual behaviours (social context, emotions involved, respecting social norms).

- A sexual obsession, like most other obsessions, can provide a sense of security for AS individuals.

Masturbation

The issue of masturbation is of utmost importance: during adolescence, auto-eroticism is the most common source of sexual satisfaction. Masturbation rates of 75% to 93% have been reported in the general population (Masters and Johnson, 1988, cited in Haracopos and Pedersen, 1999) and masturbation in itself is healthy and normal. It allows sexual tensions to be released and "can be a way of becoming more comfortable with and/or enjoying one's sexuality by getting to know and like one's body" (National Information Center for Children and Youth with Disabilities, 1992, p.14). However, masturbation can become problematic when it takes place in an inappropriate place and/or when it is accompanied by strong feelings of guilt or anxiety, in which case it is crucial that adolescents are given the opportunity to talk about it openly with a trusted person or a professional.

Teenagers with AS need to learn the difference between public places (school, store, friend's house, library, community centre, bathroom, playground) and private places (bathroom in one's home, bedroom). It is important to emphasize the conditions under which masturbation is acceptable: when individuals are alone in their room with the door closed. The message must be clear and precise to avoid misunderstandings that could lead to inappropriate behaviours and it is sometimes useful to use pictograms or key words that summarize the situation.

When masturbation becomes an individual's principal activity, the underlying motivations or possible causal factors must be explored. These may include anxiety, changes in routine, a surge in hormones, a romantic meeting, or sexual compulsion. In the latter case, adolescents must be permitted to engage in self-stimulation on a daily basis – it is normal to masturbate up to a couple of times per day.

If masturbation goes on to become detrimental to other activities, it may be necessary to expand the individual's repertoire of stimulating and interesting activities. One possible solution is to encourage them to meet new people and make new friends as a diversity of activities and encounters can create sufficient pleasure to decrease the need for auto-eroticism. Another strategy is to encourage manual activities such as drawing, painting, sculpture, writing, photography, maths, tennis, or any other activity, such as using a computer keyboard, that requires hands-on concentration. The goal is not to sublimate the sexual impulses but to diversify the individual's repertoire of stimulating activities.

The frequency of masturbation usually decreases naturally after adolescence. Sexual development should be respected and intervention strategies should help each person meet his or her needs in an acceptable and enriching manner.

Sexual assault and criminal acts

Aspies may be subject to indecent or criminal sexual behaviours such as exhibitionism, voyeurism, frotteurism, sexual assault, paedophilia, and a variety of other deviant sexual behaviours, but it is also possible that they become the perpetrators of such an assault. Below are some suggestions on how to broach the topic:

- Explain/Describe the different forms of sexual abuse to which the individual may be exposed, be it in the family, outside the family, or within a sexual relationship. The goal is to encourage him or her to feel able to express themselves about abusive situations and to develop ways to protect themselves and others.

- Discuss privacy and its boundaries, including personal examples of the kinds of rules observed within the family and between friends.

Making Waves (www.mwaves.org) is an educational programme that aims to prevent violence in sexual and romantic relationships, and in friendships. Some of its themes, outlined below, complement the activities in the sexual education programme in Part II.

- Notions of time and space: surroundings, behaviours, and individuals with whom intimate behaviour is appropriate.

- The limits of love (healthy, unhealthy, and abusive situations).

- What is dating violence?

- The cycle of violence.

- How to react to sexual assault.

- Sexuality and the law: examining different situations and asking what is acceptable or unacceptable.

- Warning signs: excessive jealousy, explosive temper, withdrawal or depression, extreme agitation, strange behaviour.

- How to prevent sexual abuse.

- How to help a friend or yourself if you recognize aggression.

As previously mentioned, aggression can fuel sexuality and generate in
ate behaviours in AS individuals. *Latent or covert aggression*, presenting as
sion or generalized distress, can be a reflection of poor socialization. *Over*
sion is expressed in *obvious*, visibly aggressive behaviours directed at ⸺.
Either type may be a result of a history of sexual abuse, imitation of observed aggressive behaviours, sexual dissatisfaction owing to the lack of a partner, experience, or stimulation, or hostility towards an individual or towards a gender
(Tremblay *et al.*, 1998).

Where an individual with AS is a victim of sexual abuse and aggression,
Hingsburger's (1995b) approach, which is based on understanding and
reducing the victim role, may be useful. Hingsburger considers sexual abuse
from the perspective of individuals with a PDD, prioritizing learning about
sexual facts, personal boundaries, the notion of consent, and openness in communication. His advocacy for sexual education and human rights opens the door
for numerous rewarding discussions for parents and professionals alike.

In some cases, inappropriate sexual behaviours take place without individuals with AS being aware of the consequences of their actions:

> A 27-year-old adult with AS was referred to me by a judge after having
> engaged in exhibitionism. One night, after having had too much to drink, he
> had decided to hitch-hike in a very busy neighbourhood. He had been
> looking for a girlfriend for several months, but none of his attempts had
> been successful. Exasperated, he impulsively pulled down his pants and
> underwear in order to get the attention of women in cars. Police arrested
> him and he had to go to court.
>
> His impulsivity interfered with his ability to think about the conse-
> quences of his actions, for which he showed great remorse. Alcohol had
> affected his judgement and sense of modesty – never before had he
> committed such an act. Initially, therapy consisted of helping him under-
> stand his actions and developing ways of controlling his impulses. He was
> made aware of the effects of alcohol and the rules regulating social conduct.
> Sessions then focused on recognizing his emotions, through physical and
> affective cues and behavioural responses, and managing them. Activities
> included in Sofronoff and Attwood's programme (2002) served as ground
> work. The development of social skills completed the therapeutic process.
>
> Given that impulsivity led to this young man's inappropriate behaviour,
> it was important to provide him with tools for preventing other impulsive
> behaviours. The work on social skills was aimed at broadening his network
> of acquaintances to encourage him to meet new people. Techniques aimed
> at managing emotions help individuals with AS to think before they act.
> Isolation sometimes leads to such an intense desire to meet a partner that
> an individual's behaviour can become impulsive and inappropriate. With
> more opportunities to make new acquaintances, individuals with AS will be
> less impulsive and desperate.

Swisher (1995) discusses treatment strategies for sex offenders. Developmental history, prior sexual experiences, substance abuse, and neurobiological factors are contributing factors in sexual offences. High levels of testosterone can be associated with increased libido and aggressiveness in offenders. Fewer criminal acts are committed by individuals with normal (70–110) intellectual quotients. Nonetheless, some criminals have distinct profiles and specific deficits (notably in terms of communication, socialization, and personality).

Sexual delinquency[1]

Papazian (unpublished, 2003) conducted a literature review on sexual delinquency in individuals with AS which concluded that the sexuality of individuals with AS generally conforms to the values and mores of the society in which they live. Few epidemiological studies have been conducted about acts of sexual delinquency in individuals with AS. Nevertheless, criminal and illegal behaviours are sometimes observed. The definition of sexual criminality varies according to country and point in time, and is usually established in law under the penal code of the state. Rape, *stricto sensu* sexual assault, sexual exhibitionism, and sexual acts with a minor are classic examples of indecent sexual acts unanimously condemned and sanctionable in many countries. Aggravating factors, or those that increase the severity of the crime, include characteristics of the victim (especially if vulnerable), perpetrator (if he or she had responsibility for or authority over the victim), modality of the offence (preceded, accompanied, or followed by acts of cruelty or torture; use of a weapon), and the outcome (death, mutilation, permanent disability).

Two issues need to be addressed. First, aggravating factors are almost always absent in sexual offences committed by individuals with AS. Second, the diagnosis of AS is often made *after* the person has committed the criminal offence, when the individual and his past history are under scrutiny.

Asperger's Syndrome and violence: Quantitative data

The prevalence of AS in the general population is underestimated, which inevitably leads to an underestimation of the number of individuals with AS who commit sexual offences. Some studies have tried to determine the relationship between AS and violence (not exclusively sexual) by attempting to establish the prevalence of the syndrome in hospitals for dangerous patients. One study, conducted by Scragg and Shah (1994) at Broadmoor Special Hospital, compared the prevalence of AS (according to Gillberg and Gillberg's (1989) criteria) in the hospital population to that of AS in the general population. Of the 392 hospital patients (all male), six were diagnosed with AS (a prevalence

---

1   This section was written in collaboration with Patrick Papazian.

rate of 1.5%). Three other, less clear, cases were added, increasing the prevalence rate to 2.3%. Although these rates are higher than that for AS in the general population, which was 0.55% at that time (Ehlers and Gillberg, 1993), it is not possible to conclude that patients with AS are more violent than the general population. Hali and Bernai (1995) argue that the difference between the samples of the two studies – in terms of country, age, and sociocultural and environmental factors – and the lack of other research done at the time make it impossible to determine whether the results are statistically significant. To date, it is therefore not possible to state categorically that individuals with AS are at greater risk of perpetrating violence than those in the general population. Despite empirical and clinical data that point to difficulties with tolerating frustration, a lack of empathy, and social difficulties (Scragg and Shah, 1994; Smith Myles and Southwick, 1999), epidemiological studies fail to conclude that individuals with AS are more likely to act on violent impulses (Ghaziuddin and Tsai, 1991).

Sexual delinquency and Asperger's Syndrome: Qualitative aspects

Several case studies describing the illegal sexual conduct of individuals with AS bear witness to their difficulties with approaching women, establishing relationships, and building intimacy. Lack of premeditation was common to all these cases. A 38-year-old man with AS who touched women sexually and engaged in frotteurism (Cooper, Mohamed and Collacott, 1993) had been unsuccessful at meeting women and, owing to his lack of empathy, failed to perceive his victims' discomfort and fear.

Mawson, Grounds and Tantam (1985) described the case of a man with AS who hit women whom he deemed insufficiently dressed, as well as crying children and barking dogs, in public places. In this case, sexuality combined with certain stimuli provoked violence, which reflected his incapacity to assimilate such auditory, visual, nonverbal, exciting, touching, or annoying stimuli. One of the most extreme cases, described by Kohn, Fahum and Ratzoni (1998), was that of a 16-year-old adolescent with AS who committed repeated sexual assault by sexually touching women whom he found attractive. During the psychiatric assessment, the adolescent showed no remorse and rationalized his actions thus: "I liked her, and I showed her…my way." Kohn *et al.* emphasize that social maladjustment, lack of empathy, and a variety of characteristics associated with AS contributed to his acting out. As such, sexual violence isn't more frequent in individuals with AS but is simply expressed according to the particularities of the syndrome, such as deficits in theory of mind, lack of sexual experience, impulsivity, difficulty expressing emotions, etc.

The case of Jeffrey Dahmer

One of the most notorious serial killers of our time, Jeffrey Dahmer, is thought to have had AS (Arturo Silva, Ferrari and Leong, 2002). In this case, the relationship between AS, psychopathology, and crimes of sexual nature can be explored from neuropsychiatric and developmental perspectives. Up until his arrest in 1991, Jeffrey Dahmer killed approximately 20 young men, engaging in acts of necrophilia and cannibalism. His cooperation with the police force and teams of psychologists and psychiatrists made it possible to collect detailed information on his family and personal history, motivations, and his interpretation of the events. One study (Arturo Silva *et al.*, 2002), published a couple of years after his death, proposed that a diagnosis of AS was probable, based upon current diagnostic criteria. The acts of necrophilia that he perpetrated seemed consistent with preoccupations that he had had since childhood. It seems that he had always been interested by the internal and external aspects of bodies, animal or human. It is believed that this quasi-obsessional interest in anatomy and collections led him to repeat his acts. According to the case study, Jeffrey Dahmer did not like killing or causing pain to his victims. The murders were justified by his wish to control his victims and find sexual satisfaction. Collecting body parts became a strong interest and a repetitive behaviour for him.

Conclusion

According to empirical data and case studies, sexual offences perpetrated by individuals with AS are no more frequent or violent than those committed by individuals in the general population. However, the context, onset, type of offence, and perception of the offence differ when it is committed by someone with AS and it is therefore crucial that preventive, educational, and therapeutic measures be made available.

Several factors can trigger or cause delinquent or criminal behaviours: substance abuse (drugs or alcohol), others' negative attitudes, past experiences, lack of judgement and empathy, and failure to understand the notion of consent. Curnoe and Langevin (2002) have proposed a variety of treatment strategies: they recommend medication (antiandrogens, Provera), group therapy, and aversion therapy for clients with PDDs. Sexual education, social skills training, and cognitive-behavioural therapy might also be considered. All treatments should consider the cognitive particularities of individuals with AS, taking into account the type of offence and the causes or triggers.

Providing the opportunity to have sexual relations with a consenting partner should be considered in cases of assault and paedophilia. However, opportunities for "supervised" sexual exchanges are not always possible (Griffiths *et al.*, 1989). Individuals with AS sometimes use the services of sex workers or surrogates to relieve their sexual needs and gain experience. This alternative must be considered carefully given the legal aspects involved.

Dennis Debbaudt commented on the scope of the dilemma that individuals with autism and AS pose for both the justice system and therapists:

> The dilemma for criminal justice professionals and the next frontier for advocacy efforts. How do we find fair justice for everyone concerned here and still address the unique needs of the person with autism? How do we advocate effectively for the offender with autism who is incarcerated? How do autism advocates begin to work with the victims? Educating law enforcement, first on the scene professionals and hospital emergency room professionals about recognition and response is the first frontier for autism advocates. Our next frontier is the rest of the criminal justice system – investigators, defense attorneys, prosecutors, judiciary and legislators, correctional professionals, social workers, forensic professionals. (Debbaudt, 2002, pp.1–2)

Chapter 3

Social skills

> Developing and maintaining satisfying interpersonal relationships are indispensable for the well-being of any person…it is quite fundamental to learn this. Who has not noticed the extent to which the smallest, most benign, daily gestures are immersed in social contexts? We are constantly interacting with our social environment…
>
> *Boisvert and Beaudry, 1985, translated by Isabelle Hénault*

This chapter proposes various theories, reflections, and tools that help polish the social, intimate, and communication skills of people with AS.

"Social aptitude" can be defined as the ability to establish relationships, maintain contact, exchange conversation in a reciprocal manner, share emotions, and develop intimacy with others. Individuals with AS have difficulty with social skills. They experience considerable discomfort which interferes with their ability to establish interpersonal relationships. Attwood (2003b) lists several characteristics related to social impairment: lack of reciprocity and maturity in relationships, limited vocabulary to describe someone's personality, adaptation strategies, limited nonverbal expression, and poor management of emotions. Some individuals with AS give greater consideration to their special interest than to interpersonal relationships. However, others show a strong interest in other people, become attracted to other teens during adolescence, and during adulthood develop a strong desire to meet a partner, share their life with someone, get married, and start a family. The image of the solitary withdrawn adolescent and adult is not accurate for everyone.

Isolation and not wanting relationships can be a choice, but individuals with AS who have the desire to establish relationships – behaviourally, emotionally, or sexually – suffer most from their limited social skills. Loneliness, depression, anxiety, frustration, and anger are frequently associated with their distress.

Although they are the cornerstones of interpersonal relationships and sexuality, the concepts of socialization and emotions cause the most confusion, fear, and misunderstanding for people with AS. Many individuals with AS avoid establishing relationships with others due to a fear of rejection that is often rooted in their sense of incompetence and lack of experience in the interpersonal and social domains.

The concept of "breaking the ice" is so terrifying for many individuals with AS that they avoid situations where they may be called upon to do so. Their past experiences play a huge role, and their pasts are often marred by negative memories. Feelings of rejection and failure, bullying and incomprehension may have resulted from social situations in the past. As a result, many people with AS avoid meeting new people and establishing social contacts, which has a direct impact on their self-esteem.

Many people with AS do suffer from loneliness and a number of them have confided that they would like to have friends, a lover, or someone with whom to share their life. Muskat (2003) described self-esteem as "the feelings and thoughts we have about ourselves, developed through experiences of relating to others, completing tasks competently, and self-direction. It includes how optimistic we are that we can succeed" (p.34). A series of exercises, activities, and tools are included in the sociosexual education programme in Part 2 of this book to increase the sense of control and self-esteem of individuals with AS. Positive social experiences strengthen self-confidence and act as powerful reinforcers. The exercises allow people to question and position themselves in a variety of situations, learn about the rules of communication, define intimacy, and decode nonverbal language. One young adult with AS told me:

> Even if I'm satisfied with the way that some encounters have gone, I'm still afraid to make the first move. I have been disappointed so many times that I am sometimes resigned to the idea that I will spend my life alone. And yet, I like the company of others, but I always expect failure. I need to replace my bad experiences with new ones. I need to explore other kinds of human relationships. This takes a lot of energy, but it's worth it.

The "butterflies in the stomach" associated with new relationships (both friendship and romantic) can take on totally different proportions. In his book *Freaks, Geeks and Asperger Syndrome* (2002), Luke Jackson describes his first apprehensions in the context of relationships:

> I never asked anyone out in my entire life, although I have wanted to quite a few times. Perhaps by the time of publication this may have changed, but even if that is so, I find it very hard to envisage me turning into some kind of Casanova! (p.170)

The book describes his experience of adolescence and AS, and lists a variety of practical tips for first dates by referring to the "Dating Game" (p.176). There is nothing more imprecise or unpredictable than first dates. An "instruction manual" can therefore be quite helpful. With time and practice, spontaneity develops. Below are some tools that will help people with AS "break the ice" and develop better social skills.

Tools to improve social skills

The goal of social skills training is to polish and expand the adaptive behaviour repertoire of individuals with AS. There is a substantial relationship between interpersonal skills and sexuality: apart from self-stimulation, sexual behaviours are experienced and shared with other people. Verbal and nonverbal communication are important from the start in order to bring people together, express desires, feelings, and meet again. Before any of this can happen, some indispensable basic skills are required.

Social and interpersonal skills training is extremely valuable for the AS population. In addition to improving the quality of social interactions, intervention programmes teach new behaviours and how to integrate them into participants' daily lives. Attwood and Gray (1999a) tackle friendship skills with strategies adapted to the specific needs of people with AS. Introduction skills (joining a group, introducing oneself, greeting others) are at the basis of all interactions. Social skills training programmes are only one of several kinds of intervention, from group activities to cognitive behaviour therapy.

During a social skills training programme, participants engage in and complete a variety of exercises each week. The group format helps foster social learning (learning through observing others). Over the course of the socio-sexual education programme presented in Part 2 of this book, reciprocity among participants grows and some discover shared interests, the basis of any friendship (Hénault *et al.*, 2003). During the first meetings, participants tend to remain isolated and do not really interact much with one another. The activities in the subsequent workshops enhance participants' conversation skills. Communication and intimacy skills are also improved. Attwood and Gray (1999a) developed the Friendship Skills Observation Checklist specifically for people with AS in order to assess progressive gains in basic skills, which makes it possible to follow the evolution of each participant's skills each week. The most recent version of the Friendship Skills Observation Checklist (Attwood and Gray, 1999a) is now known as the Indices of Friendship Observation Schedule (Attwood, 2003c) and is available at *www.tonyattwood.com.au* under "Tony's publications".

Attwood and Gray's 1999 version of the observation schedule includes 14 general social skills subdivided into 24 behaviours (Attwood and Gray, 1999a). Each interpersonal skill is accompanied by a descriptor that defines its specific content and is rated along a five-point Likert scale where "1" indicates that the participant exhibits less than 10% of the skill observed, "3" represents 50%, and "5" represents more than 90% . It is completed by an outside observer, such as a teacher or group leader, and completing it makes it possible for the frequency and proportion of behaviours that each individual with AS engages in to be observed. The Friendship Skills Observation Checklist (Attwood and Gray, 1999a) can be used throughout the programme as a *post hoc* measure.

Ouellet and L'Abbé's (1986) social skills programme is explicit about the importance of socialization. The authors propose exercises (role-playing different situations, vignettes) based on five categories of social skills. The first category consists of "basic skills" such as caring for one's appearance, listening, participating in a conversation, saying thank you, and giving a compliment. The second category deals with "advanced skills" such as apologizing, giving instructions, offering and asking for help, sharing, and problem-solving. The third category consists of "expression of feelings": activities first identify one's own emotions and those of others, then target how to respond to teasing and to failure. The fourth category deals with "assertiveness training". Activities are focused on negotiation, refusal, valuing one's rights and opinions, and managing aggression. The last category addresses issues around the topic of "respect". Role-playing situations focus on being attentive to others, respecting authority and rules, and identifying inappropriate touch. Overall, this programme covers many skills relevant to the interpersonal development of individuals with AS.

Visual contact

Maintaining visual contact, characterized by the ability to read facial expressions and to show interest in others, is an important communication skill. It requires serious concentration from individuals with AS because some have difficulty detecting and analysing verbal and nonverbal stimuli. Some Aspies avoid eye contact with other people in order to concentrate and to pay attention to what is being said. This behaviour is unfortunately often interpreted by others as lack of interest. Individuals with AS need to develop strategies to help them maintain a minimum of visual contact. This is especially important in romantic relationships. A social education programme for young people with AS in New Jersey, the Friendship Club, offers social skills training that focuses specifically on the development of visual contact (Graham, 2003).

Affective behaviours

Hugs are manifestations of love, affection, compassion, and joy; they are not only pleasant, but necessary. Scientists all around the world have shown that hugs are essential to our physical and emotional well-being. Keating (1994) explores the questions of how we express affection to others and what kind of hug expresses which emotion in *The Little Book of Big Hugs*, using fifty or so pictures of bears (symbolizing affection) to illustrate different kinds of hugs and their meanings. Simple and practical, this little book can be particularly useful and entertaining for young people with AS who frequently lack reference points for the use of intimate gestures. They can also use this book to decode and imitate affectionate behaviour when they are learning about appropriate intimate behaviours.

Communication

Communication is composed of verbal and nonverbal language. The majority of individuals with AS possess language skills, but their communication skills are usually poor. Verbal exchanges only account for about 30% of communication whereas nonverbal language makes up 70%.

Verbal communication

Verbal communication is the act of conveying one's meaning to another person using words, holding a conversation. Attwood (2003b) lists the pragmatic aspects of conversation for people with AS since they experience difficulties including lack of reciprocity, inappropriate comments, monologues, literal interpretations, mimicry, excessive technical details, idiosyncrasies and neologisms, inappropriate volume of speech, inappropriate voicing of thoughts, and hypersensitive hearing. Communication skills can be taught by encouraging individuals with AS to participate in activities that will enable them to practise their skills, for example asking for directions, starting and holding a conversation, giving a compliment, giving their opinion on something, or talking about plans for the weekend. Individual and group interventions can be adapted to communication exercises.

The four main principles of communication that make it possible to have a good conversation with someone are: "I express myself", "I listen", "I verify", and "I consider the other person" (Boisvert and Beaudry, 1985).

1. *I express myself.* I say what I think and feel in a clear, precise, and brief manner. I express what I feel in a non-accusing but direct and constructive way. I express my requests in a positive way and I do not go off-topic (by bringing up old discussions or unrelated content such as my specific interest). Finally, I respect the other person; I avoid making insults and disparaging remarks. The discussion must always be respectful.

2. *I listen.* I let the other person talk and I listen actively (by paying attention to the discussion).

3. *I verify.* To avoid misunderstandings, I verify that I understood properly what the other person was saying (by reformulating it in my own words). I also make sure that the other person understood what I said. Since I can't read the other person's mind and they can't read mine, I check that the other person thinks and feels what I

think (for example, I can start a sentence by saying "Do you mean that...").

4. *I consider the other person.* I respect the other person. I notice their positive behaviours (efforts made to express themselves, openness to the discussion, how well they listen, etc.). When I agree with the other person, I tell them honestly (for example, "I agree with what you just said..."). Continually disagreeing with someone leads to misunderstandings. If I don't agree, I can still recognize the value of the other's point of view (for example, "Even if I don't agree with what you just said, I respect your opinion on...").

Boisvert and Beaudry (1985) suggest practical exercises and role-play situations for individuals with AS. Role-playing and rehearsal strategies help address these principles of verbal communication. These can take place in small groups or with an individual participant and should take examples of conversations from daily life – with peers, family members, shopkeepers, and so on – to help the person with AS explore communication and analyse the presence or absence of the four principles listed above. Elements of a discussion can be analysed by making audio recordings of some of these conversations. Participants should be encouraged to apply what they have learned to other situations, through role-play in the group or practising with friends or family members. They should be encouraged to initiate a conversation with someone they know. It is important to encourage all attempts: resistance is often due to a sense of inadequacy and fear of rejection, and people with AS will resist less if they have gained confidence from positive experiences.

Nonverbal communication

Nonverbal language is the most important component of communication and includes facial expressions, emotions, gestures, body language, and visual contact. Muskat (2003) discussed the difficulties that people with AS have with social competence and the need to help them understand their environment and interactions with others better. Modelling, practical rehearsal strategies, and positive reinforcement help individuals with AS learn practically how to communicate with and decode nonverbal language.

A useful exercise for practising nonverbal communication is to reproduce the contents of a vignette using gestures (no words allowed!). Examples include "I feel good with you", "I'm nervous because I have to meet my boss", "I lost my dog and it makes me sad", or "I am preoccupied today; I need to make an important decision". Further vignettes can be found in Lemay's (1996) education programme. Elements from daily life are taken up and summarized in short phrases that must then be mimed nonverbally, and the vignettes can be adapted to the experiences of those participating in the activity. Concrete examples of everyday situations include "I am happy when I play on the computer", "I am nervous about meeting the other students in my class" or "I am angry because my brother broke my favourite game". Another exercise involves rehearsing situations with intimate and emotional context, and one such exercise is integrated into the sociosexual education programme (see Workshop 12).

It is possible to learn to decode nonverbal language using scenes where an interaction is occurring on television or in movie clips. You should start with simple interactions (between two people) and turn off the volume so that the individual with AS can decode the meaning of the nonverbal communication they see during the interaction. The following questions can accompany the exercise:

- What is happening?

- What message(s) is/are transmitted by which character?

- What emotion(s) is/are expressed?

- What gestures express the emotion, action, or message?

Showing several sequences to the individual with AS and repeating the exercise are of considerable value; magazine pictures could also be used. When individuals have acquired a certain level of comprehension and they feel sufficiently comfortable, they can act out the scene and mime its nonverbal content. Rehearsal should take place with two people at first; more complex interactions should be introduced gradually by adding characters.

Motor abilities are also used during role-play situations. Fine motor skills (movement of small muscles, e.g. fingers to grasp) and gross motor skills (movement of larger muscles requiring different levels of control, e.g. whole arm) and coordination are involved in nonverbal communication. Awareness of one's body in space can also be taught, in particular with individuals who tend to "crowd" people in conversation. The goal is to integrate visual environmental cues. Examples from daily life can serve as starting points for all these exercises.

Emotions

The diagnostic criteria that surround AS (APA, 1994; WHO, 1993) attest to the difficulties people with AS have in maintaining eye contact and decoding nonverbal language. Workshops on emotions and theory of mind (Hénault *et al.*, 2003) allow participants to work on these skills by role-playing and using the *Mind-Reading* and *Gaining Face* software (Baron-Cohen *et al.*, 2004; Team Asperger, 2000). Individuals with AS have difficulty interpreting emotions because they focus on the details (such as eyebrows, eyes, mouth, etc.) of the human face without having a complete picture of the face. It takes them a long time to observe the whole face and the task often becomes laborious as facial expressions change rapidly. Individuals with AS don't have time to decode one emotion before it is replaced by another. This may lead to a fixed gaze (while concentrating on the task of analysing the details and emotions of the face) or avoidance of eye contact (due to information overload).

Certain behaviours (handshakes, winks, smiles, etc.) can replace staring and the decoding difficulties encountered, and there are numerous exercises, from role play to interpreting body language, that enable people with AS to increase the movement in their gaze. Exercises for emotions are presented in the sociosexual skills education programme in this book (Workshops 6 and 12).

Activities in "A cognitive behaviour therapy intervention for anxiety in children with Asperger's Syndrome" (Sofronoff and Attwood, 2002) help individuals with AS improve their emotion recognition and management skills. Group activities are presented in a series of sessions and include a description of emotions, a journal, questionnaires, games, thought-provoking exercises, and a project on emotions. The Biotouch Interactive Mood Light (Sharper Image Design, 1999) complements the programme. This device allows internal physical reactions (e.g., "I feel nervous") to be associated with colours. Several lights go off when fingers are placed on sensors. Yellow and green lights are associated with calm or sadness whereas orange and red lights are signs of activity (positive: excited, dynamic; or negative: anger or anxiety). Individuals with AS can learn to identify their emotional states and use relaxation techniques. For example, someone who is anxious activates red lights when he places his fingers on the device. He can then consult a sheet where a range of practical tips are listed next to each circle of colour. Next to the red circle, the following tips are listed: "Take 5 deep breaths, think about my specific interest, imagine myself somewhere in particular, retire to a quiet spot, go for a walk, write in my journal, take a bath, speak to a friend".

If the person is calm (yellow light), she can pursue her activities and the counsellor can reinforce the behaviour (congratulate, reward, offer a treat, etc.). If she is sad (orange light), she can consult a list of related activities, such as: "Talk about my feelings to someone, cry, draw, write in my journal, rest, read, call a friend and explain what is going on, practise an activity related to my specific interest". Tips can be adapted to each individual in order to help them manage their anxiety. Activities and ideas should accompany the different categories of emotion. With training and practice, individuals with AS can use the mood light independently and apply the suggestions as needed as part of their progress towards autonomy.

Automatic thoughts

Automatic negative thoughts have a considerable impact on behaviour and self-confidence. They are spontaneous and recurrent and accompany stressful and difficult situations. Automatic thoughts cause physiological activity (stress,

✔

1. Situation	2. Behaviours	3. Sensations	4. Emotions
What is the situation? Where? When? With whom? What is happening?	What are my actions? Describe my behaviours.	What are my physical sensations? • Positive • Negative	What am I feeling? What are my emotions, feelings, moods? Rate them on a scale of 1 (very negative) to 10 (very positive).
5. Automatic thoughts/images What are my spontaneous thoughts? My negative thoughts?	**6. Facts that support the automatic thoughts** My past experiences. What makes me believe my automatic thoughts?	**7. Facts that contradict the automatic thoughts** Facts that are different from the preceding ones. Experiences that are more positive.	**8. Alternative realistic thoughts** What could I tell myself that is more realistic? My positive and realistic thoughts.

9. I reassess my affective state and I note changes in my behaviour
How do I feel now? Rates positive emotions on a scale of 1 (very negative) to 10 (very positive).
Are my sensations more positive than negative? What are my behaviours now?

Figure 3.1 Self-monitoring sheet (adapted from Lazarus, 1976)

1. Situation	2. Behaviour	3. Sensations	4. Emotions
I'm invited to a party. I know two people who will be there. I must take public transport. I have nothing else planned for the evening.	I look for my map of the city. I must have a shower and iron my clothes. I telephone to confirm that I will attend. I plan my schedule for the evening: departure, trip, and return.	I feel nervous, I'm trembling, and my breathing is shallow. I feel perturbed because I rarely attend parties like this.	I'm worried because I hope that all will go well tonight. I'm afraid of missing the bus and of being late. I'm also anxious because I don't know a lot of the people who will be there tonight. My rating of the intensity of these feelings is 8/10, which is high.
5. Automatic thoughts/images	6. Facts that support the automatic thoughts	7. Facts that contradict the automatic thoughts	8. Alternative realistic thoughts
Everyone will see that I'm nervous. Once again, I'll be alone in my corner. What if the two people that I know decide not to go? I don't know what to wear. I have to be courteous with the girls and not make any negative comments. I have to make conversation.	I didn't speak to anyone the last time that I went to a party. I also spilled my drink on a girl's skirt and had to apologize. I would have preferred to be at my computer.	This time I know two people who seem quite nice. I won't be alone and I feel like meeting girls. At the last party, a pretty girl told me "See you soon, I hope" – maybe she'd like to see me again? After all, it's Saturday night.	This might give me the opportunity to see that girl again. I could wear my new shirt, it's not bad. I'm going and who knows? I may have fun. I'll come home early. I feel like getting out of the house. I'm capable of listening to a conversation. If I find it difficult, I can take a break (outside). I must take the initiative.

9. I reassess my affective state and I note changes in my behaviour
I'm going and I'm happy about my decision. I feel calmer and more relaxed. Even though I know that I will be nervous, I'll take three deep breaths and I'll think of the positive things. I'm organizing myself and I'll be on time. I'm taking the initiative and I'm proud of myself. I can come home whenever I want. I rate my feelings as 4/10, which is less intense and problematic.

Figure 3.2 Example of a completed self-monitoring sheet (adapted from Lazarus, 1976)

anxiety, tension etc.) and provoke emotions (fear, sadness, incompetence, etc.). Self-monitoring can help individuals to deal with these thoughts. It allows individuals to analyse difficult situations, factors which maintain automatic thought (e.g. stress, lack of confidence, etc.), and the behavioural consequences.

Easy-to-use self-monitoring sheets based on cognitive theories can be useful (adapted from Lazarus, 1976; see Figures 3.1 and 3.2). The observation sheet (Figure 3.1) can be completed alone or with the help of a counsellor (see the example in Figure 3.2). The goal is to help individuals with AS modify their thoughts and behaviours, helping them face situations in a more realistic and positive manner. They should take a specific situation and complete the nine boxes, answering the questions with that situation in mind. Examples of situations that could be explored in this way are social outings, dates, misunderstandings, sexual desire towards someone, a new job, or any other stressful situation. Figure 3.2 illustrates the automatic thoughts that might accompany an invita-

ASPERGER'S SYNDROME AND SEXUALITY

tion to a social outing. Exploring alternatives to these negative thoughts will help individuals have a more appropriate and positive view of the situation. In consequence, physiological activity will decrease and emotions will be less negative. Regular practice and use of this tool will increase its effectiveness.

Theory of mind

"Theory of mind" is the capacity to attribute mental states to oneself and others. This capacity for "meta-representation" is usually achieved around the age of four years but is delayed in individuals with AS (Tréhin, 1999). Even if they have no intellectual disability, individuals with AS will only develop theory of mind at around eight years of age (Poirier, 1998). Several neurological explanations have been proposed (Adolphs, Sears and Piven, 2001; Brent *et al.*, 2001). One explanation is that individuals with AS don't use the same part of the brain as neurotypicals for tasks related to facial recognition and social situations. Functional magnetic resonance imagery (fMRI) has made it possible to detect different activation patterns in certain parts of the frontal lobe and amygdala. Young (2001) reviewed Brent *et al.*'s work and noted that recognition of social indicators activate the parts of the brain responsible for general intelligence and cognitive problem-solving in individuals with AS. Individuals in the general population show a very different pattern of activation. These results suggest that dysfunction of the amygdala could be responsible for errors in social judgement, leading to inappropriate behaviours. Similarly, Channon *et al.* (2001) noted that subjects with AS had difficulty completing problem-solving tasks and those involving social conflict. Their responses were quite different to those usually reported among the general population. Other explanations include poor central coherence and lack of cognitive flexibility.

The concept of "emotional intelligence" is defined as the capacity to recognize one's emotions, manage emotions so that they are appropriate to a given situation, recognize others' emotions, and cope with interpersonal relationships (Hess, 1998). Sustained training to develop emotional intelligence in people with AS must first focus on the essentials – recognizing anger, joy, sadness and, over time, a wider and more subtle repertoire of emotions – and by doing so reduce the flood of information that accompanies facial decoding. Activities found in *Teaching Children with Autism to Mind-read* (Howlin, Baron-Cohen and Hadwin, 1999) help reduce these difficulties by teaching theory of mind to young people with AS. In addition, the *Mind-Reading* software (Baron-Cohen *et al.*, 2004), an interactive educational tool, presents a full range of emotions, situations involving verbal and nonverbal communication, and theory of mind.

Conclusion

In Chapter 3 we have looked at some tools and interventions which complement the sexual education programme in the second part of this book. It is always possible to add some social skills exercises from these tools to many of the topics addressed in the programme (e.g. those on love and friendship; sexual relations and sexual behaviours; emotions; sexuality; sexism; managing emotions, theory of mind, and intimacy). Interventions aimed at improving social competency will improve interpersonal relationships. The goal is to allow individuals with AS to explore and manage their emotions, decode basic nonverbal messages, and understand social interactions better. They will consequently be able to identify emotions such as anxiety, aggression, and withdrawal and will gradually be able to see the relationship between social situations, their thoughts, feelings, and behaviours. Developing social skills improves the capacity to establish and maintain social relationships and take the initiative, which has a direct impact on self-esteem (Muskat, 2003).

Chapter 4

Sexual diversity and gender identity

A veritable "empire of the sexes" (Dorais, 1999) has invaded the popular culture of most Western societies. Sexuality is dominated by marked opposites; standards, norms, and gender definitions are all seen in terms of "male" or "female". Is sexuality not composed of personal, cultural, and historical variations? Nowadays, social norms take precedence over sexual diversity, which is often viewed as perverse. However, some people fail to conform to these established norms, for example effeminate boys, masculine girls, and androgynous, transsexual, intersex, or transvestite individuals.

Empirical studies, clinical observations, and Internet discussion groups make it possible to establish a link between gender identity (the subjective sense of being male or female), sexual diversity, and AS. This chapter will therefore explore an aspect of sexuality in individuals with AS that affects quite a number of people but is rarely discussed.

Sexual diversity

The results of a study of 28 adults with AS described in the Appendix showed that the participants were generally in harmony with their sense of being male or female, and their scores for identifying with their sexual roles were equivalent to those of the general population. The gender identities of the participants were firmly anchored in their personalities and surprisingly unaffected by social norms.

The responses also showed an openness towards sexual diversity. When asked to comment on the notion of sexual diversity, one adult with AS stated:

> I can only speak from experience, but for me, I'm less inclined to be bound to traditional relationship structures, and more inclined to ask what is hurtful vs. healthy in an objective sense, rather than assume that a "marriage-like" monogamous pairing is the only valid relationship model.

We are male or female, masculine or feminine, homosexual or heterosexual. But why these eternal oppositions? Dorais (1999) transcends these dualities and explores the complexity of the human being. His provocative ideas have challenged traditional notions of sexuality for more than 20 years. His *Éloge de la diversité sexuelle* denounces fundamentalism in sexuality. His reflections stem from his clinical and educational experience in social work, and he is an advocate for all of those who do not fit into society's preconceived notions of what is "normal". He has worked closely with, and collected testimonies from, individuals who have suffered due to their sexual "difference".

The AS population is different from the general population in its very nature, and this difference is experienced in many areas, including at the level of sexual diversity. According to Dorais (1999, cited in Hénault, 2000, p.55):

> Never have the body and physical appearance been as valued…and yet, more and more people experience sexual ambiguity. These are feminine boys, masculine girls, androgynes, transvestites, transsexuals, hermaphrodites and all those for whom identity is much more than a question of norms. Individuals take precedence, with their stories, experiences, and particularities. Why try to trap them into any sexual standard? [Translated by Isabelle Hénault.]

His message is that sexual diversity should be acknowledged and welcomed. In order to do this, we must take three elements into account: sexual identity (biological sex), gender identity (the sense of being male or female), and eroticism (sexual preference). Dorais emphasizes the need to stop associating diversity with perversity.

Distinctions must be made between individuals who suffer due to their difference and those who play with diversity, as in the case of androgynes and transvestites who put on a show (otherwise known as "drag queens"). As the expression of both sexes, androgyny is fascinating and more or less socially acceptable. Transvestites are seen as "stars of the stage" but they, as well as men who dress as women all the time, find that their ambiguity is not well tolerated once the show is over, and their daily lives are filled with suffering. They provoke a variety of reactions; they both fascinate and disturb and, according to Dorais, attraction and repulsion are different sides of the same coin. Such a transgression of rules is destabilizing for a purist society. Some adults manage to defend their rights, but this is rarely the case for adolescents – questions about sexual identity begin at that age.

The biological sex of a child is the first thing to be established at birth: "it's a boy" or "it's a girl". Children are exposed to gender categories from an early age, but sexual identity is experienced differently by some, including a proportion of individuals with AS, as evidence from Internet discussion groups and interviews with adolescents and adults demonstrate.

A 17-year-old with AS decided to change his name to give it a feminine connotation. He started to answer to the name Patricia. He let his hair grow, wore nail polish and a bra that he stole from his mother. His parents tolerated his behaviour at home but forbade it at school or during outings. His male characteristics caused him distress. He shaved twice a day and tried to hide his genitals with loose clothing.

This lasted for close to two years, during which Patricia's anxiety was palpable. There were numerous conflicts at home and his parents didn't know how to deal with the situation. When they questioned him about his change in gender identity, Patricia responded rationally that he was a girl and that was why he behaved in that way.

One day, Patricia told his mother that he would now answer to the name of Patrick (his real name). His mother was stunned and during the discussion that ensued, Patrick told her for the first time what pushed him to become Patricia. He didn't accept his diagnosis of AS. His father also had difficulty accepting the situation and sometimes told him to "stop acting retarded". In an attempt to be accepted, he decided to be totally different and become someone else. He told himself: "I am a boy with AS. If I'm a girl, I won't have AS any more." His name change marked this decision.

Patrick's case is not uncommon. Adolescents with AS who have difficulty accepting their diagnosis may react in unexpected ways, and professionals must therefore be sensitive when giving and discussing a diagnosis. Attwood (2003b) recommends that it be explained to young people by referring to AS as a "sixth sense" based on their unique qualities. He and Carol Gray have developed criteria based on the strengths and aptitudes of AS rather than the deficits (Attwood and Gray, 1999b). Their useful resource also suggests tools to help newly diagnosed individuals with any difficulties they may have with the diagnosis (books, programmes, activities, etc.). Attwood (2003b) lists a variety of famous people suspected of having AS: this is a good starting-point for an exploration of the advantages of AS.

If someone displays drastic and sudden changes in their sexual orientation or behaviour, a reaction to a situation or state is usually indicated – Patrick is a good example. In contrast, the gradual but sustained development of different sexual behaviours, can be due to changes in personality.

Transvestic and fetishistic behaviours have been observed in the Asperger population. "Transvestism" is defined as the marked and persistent presence of sexual desires, fantasies, and behaviour related to seeking and obtaining sexual gratification by wearing opposite sex clothing and/or accessories (Département de Sexologie, 1996). Some women report that their partners with AS experience periods of transvestism. Despite taboos and fear of judgement, these women have talked about their intimate experiences and how sexual diversity has affected their sexual lives. The partner with AS explores feminine clothing and accessories in order to add to the couple's sexual repertoire. Free from taboo, they play around with the concept of gender.

Clothing worn by the opposite sex may also hold a particular meaning that is not connected with the erotic. A man with AS once told me that he felt more comfortable wearing his wife's clothes because this made the difference between them (AS versus neurotypical) disappear. An adolescent dressed like his older sister in order to look like her friends so that he could play with and feel accepted by them. Another wore girls' underwear in order to resemble the counsellors who took care of him: interpersonal contact was easier for him if he was the "same sex" as them. Transvestism can be used to do away with feelings of difference and help feel accepted by peers. When teachers, youth workers, and caretakers are all women, males with AS may wish to "become" like those who accept them, namely women. Some say that they feel more acceptance for their transvestism than their AS.

Others develop transvestite fetishes. Charles de Brosses introduced the term *fétiche* in 1760 in his article "Les Dieux Fétiches". The word "fetish" originates from the Portuguese word *feitico*, which refers to artificial or charmed things. It took more than 100 years for the notion of fetishism to be introduced in sexology. Alfred Binet (1887) described sexual fetishism as the tendency to objectify, glorify, and deify an object or body part above and beyond any mere human being. Sexual excitement is procured from inanimate objects, nonsexual body parts, or the physical or psychological particularities of an individual, and this becomes the *sine qua non* for sexual pleasure. It is important not to confuse fetishism with sexual, erotic, or aesthetic preferences. It is perfectly normal to be attracted to a specific type of person or nationality or to prefer a particular body shape.

There are three categories of sexual fetishism. *Non-transvestic fetishism* can be described as sexual excitement procured by a fetish (body part, object, characteristic of a person). *Transvestic fetishism* involves cross-dressing for the purpose of sexual excitement; the cross-dressing is usually partial (accessories, stockings, lingerie) here. Finally, *sado-masochistic fetishism* can lead to sadistic or masochistic behaviours that involve varying levels of sexual aggression.

In terms of popular psychology, fetishism is a way of increasing an individual or a couple's sexual excitement. Sexual accessories, erotic material, and fantasies should in no way be considered deviant or perverse. For some, having recourse to a fetish makes sexual arousal more concrete. Pleasure is obtained from seeing and touching the fetishistic object. It is therefore easier for the individual to concentrate on obtaining pleasure. One woman with AS told me that it was easier for her to view the sexual act as a means of obtaining pleasure from physical sensations and erotic objects. "My behaviour may seem genitally focused and even animalistic because my pleasure doesn't come from an emotional or interpersonal exchange."

Sexual orientation

Sexual orientation is independent of gender identity. Sexual orientation is defined by sexual preference (homosexual, bisexual, or heterosexual). "Homosexuality" can be described as having sexual fantasies, desires, and behaviours directed to individuals of the same sex (Département de Sexologie, 1996). "Heterosexuality" involves the opposite sex. "Bisexuality" can be defined as the coexistence of homo- and heterosexual desires and behaviours, with a preferred orientation.

The sense of being male or female should not influence sexual orientation. Why should a lesbian not be feminine? Why shouldn't a gay man be masculine in the same way as a "straight" man? Lack of understanding and taboos lead to ideas such as "lesbians must be masculine-looking" or "someone must always take on the role of the male or female partner in a homosexual relationship". Such stereotypes only serve to increase society's resistance to sexual diversity.

Several clinicians and researchers have recently become interested in the relationship between sexual orientation, autism, and AS. One preconceived notion is that individuals with AS are asexual, void of sexual desire, sexual needs, or sexual behaviour. When asked "Do you think that people with AS are asexual or is this more of a social prejudice?" one individual with AS responded:

> I do know of some AS people who are largely asexual, but the majority I know have some interest in sex. I suspect there may be a couple of mechanisms at play here. One is social prejudice (including the simple fact that asexuality is "easier" to handle when the traditional audience has been parents with kids). Another could be that some people are tactile defensive, which may make sex unpleasant for them, even though they otherwise have sexual interests. Like any segment of population, there is diversity, and there are a lot of people with AS who are anything BUT asexual.

In some cases, asexuality is an integral part of the process of self-identification, but in others it is a temporary state that leads to exploration and gender transition (Israel and Tarver, 1997). The sexual identity and orientation of individuals with AS is often idiosyncratic and free of the taboos that surround gender diversity. One adult with AS explained: "I am attracted first and foremost to the person, their qualities, and personality. Their being a man or a woman is not important to me." This is why some individuals with AS consider themselves to be bisexual, homosexual, or even ambisexual.

To date, no empirical data are available on the prevalence of homosexuality among people with AS. However, for several reasons, I suspect that the prevalence rate is high. Like everyone else, individuals with AS are strongly affected by their environment and prior sexual experiences. First sexual experiences, behaviours, and desires can be oriented to those in the immediate environment, and due to the high male:female ratio in the AS population, there is a greater chance for a male with AS to be surrounded by other males. Another factor is attraction to what is similar: for some people it may be less intimidating to establish an intimate/sexual relationship with someone who is "similar" to them. Prior sexual experiences are also important, and individuals with AS, for whom repetition and routine are important elements of the behavioural repertoire, are likely to repeat previously satisfying experiences, be they homo-, bi- or hetero-sexual.

Some heterosexual men with AS have "effeminate" traits or characteristics. Their "effeminate" mannerisms, "camp" behaviour, and choice of clothing may give the superficial impression of homosexuality. Individuals with AS pay little attention to this kind of stereotype and cliché, which is why their behaviour is often misinterpreted.

Other individuals with AS are quite categorical about their sexual orientation and can express themselves very strongly.

> Carl, a 20-year-old with AS, was quite preoccupied with his image. He wished to express his masculinity in such a way as to be attractive to young women. He imitated the behaviour of popular male movie stars and models. He worked out, didn't shave, and wore clothing that drew attention to his muscles.

For Carl, taking on "superficial" male attributes is an expression of his attraction towards women and therefore, like other young men, Carl takes care in his masculine appearance. However, if people are judged only according to how they look and what they wear, the result may be confusing, as in the following example.

> Lili had just celebrated her 18th birthday. She had been waiting impatiently for this moment because it signified that she could freely express her sexual orientation and desires. In order to express her desire for women, Lili got dressed in an ultra-feminine manner (mini-skirt, high heels, tight camisole, heavy make-up) and went out to a bar. As can be expected, more men than women were attracted to her and the evening ended in failure when a man asked her to spend the night with him.

It was logical for Lili to express her femininity in order to attract women because she believed that we are attracted to what is similar to us. However, others interpreted her intent quite differently. Cases like this demonstrate that the image and sexual preferences of individuals with AS can frequently be misunderstood. Some try to look and behave like stereotypes of men and women because their interpretation of these roles is very literal. However, sexual identity is a set of characteristics that go beyond outward appearances.

Conversely, people with AS may also have a very flexible attitude to image and sexual orientation. They may be attracted to a *person*, regardless of their gender. Some individuals with AS who have had male and female partners do not consider themselves as bisexual, but as ambisexual. "Ambisexuality" can be defined as the simultaneous or successive *preference-free* coexistence of homosexual and heterosexual behaviour, where fantasy is centred on the sexual situation and not the gender of the partner (Département de Sexologie, 1996). Clearly, individuals with AS can express their sexuality in a variety of ways.

The diagnosis of autism or AS can eclipse those issues encountered that are related to sexual orientation, and for many young people a double diagnosis (sexual orientation and AS) only serves to complicate matters. Several individuals have lived their lives as homosexual or bisexual without being diagnosed with AS, and for some, despite being considered strange or different, this has eased their lives. Below are two comments of adults with autism and AS on sexual orientation:

> At school, I used a different strategy, and completely denied my gay feelings. Being "geeky" was enough to keep my profile low so that my sexuality wasn't really questioned. Becoming "asexual" wasn't an option for me, as it was quite obvious to me that I wasn't.

> As for autistic sexuality – hypersensitivity and social alienation definitely affect sexuality. I am not sure if homosexuality, the kind that makes people identify with it instead of just doing it when their wives/husbands are away, is on the spectrum or whether ACs [autistic people] are more likely to be open minded.

A sexually repressed childhood can amplify symptoms of autism because sexual repression may affect the individual's openness to the world, interpersonal relationships, expression of emotion, and communication. These are the difficulties that one sexually diverse adult with AS had to surmount:

> He discovered his homosexuality but because he and others around him had such difficulties dealing with and accepting his AS, he suppressed his sexual desires and fantasies to the point that he was no longer conscious of them. Like many others, he thought for a long time that he was the only one to experience this duality (AS and homosexuality). Low self-esteem and high levels of stress also contributed to his difficulties. Through his experiences in support groups and Internet discussions, he finally realized that "I am just one of the many people trying to find their place in the world".

Internet discussion groups allow individuals with AS to interact with many people and to gain self-confidence by discussing intimate topics. Gay and bisexual adults with autism and AS have come together in order to obtain recognition, support, and professional services adapted to their needs. These information and support groups allow members to share their experiences and learn from one another. Some denounce the silence of professionals who ignore their condition or label them as "queer" (having a non-mainstream, different sexuality). Support is crucial given that coming to terms with sexual orientation can be quite painful. Self-acceptance and self-esteem develop through respectful reflections and exchanges and support groups can provide substantial help in doing this. The subject can also be further addressed in therapy. Information and sexual education are also important, and useful exercises are presented in the Sexual Education Programme in Part Two (Workshop 8).

Gender identity

"Gender identity", the sense of being male or female, can be defined as the profound sense of individuation, differentiation, and belonging to a biological sex that gradually forms during an individual's psychosexual development (Département de Sexologie, 1996). Gender identity can be expressed in a variety of ways, and where it differs from sexual identity it may take the form of, for example, transvestism and transsexualism.

According to the *Lexique des termes sexologiques* (Département de Sexologie, 1996), transvestism is not a gender identity disorder. As we discussed earlier in this chapter, cross-dressing can serve more than sexual needs and can be about identification with the opposite sex. The sense of belonging to the opposite sex and discomfort with one's anatomical sex can sometimes lead to transsexuality and surgery. "Transsexualism" can be defined as the wish for the permanent transformation of one's genitals in order to identify with the opposite sex; it is found in approximately one man in 20,000 and one woman in 50,000. The DSM-IV (APA, 1994) considers transsexualism to be a disorder of gender identity. Israel and Tarver (1997) claim "There is no reason why psychiatrists and other mental health professionals cannot be charged with the responsibility of recognizing gender identity issues without the necessity of labelling them as disorders" (p.25). Physical transformation is sometimes the only way in which gender identity distress and its accompanying symptoms, including low self-esteem, social isolation, psychological distress, and depression, can be relieved (Gale, 2001).

Sexual orientation is not involved in gender identity disorder: in fact, sexual preference (for men or women) must always be identified separately. Moebius (1998) has suggested that gender identity disorder is one way in which homosexuality first manifests itself and Gale (2001) supports this, finding that close to 75% of boys with gender identity disorder are homosexual or bisexual. Zucker and Bradley (1995) (as cited in Moebius, 1998), on the other hand, believe that, even though some individuals with gender identity disorder have a homosexual orientation, most homosexuals do not have gender identity concerns during their childhood. They suggest several factors that can contribute to gender identity disorders. Children can identify with the opposite sex if that sex is perceived as reassuring or superior. Behaving like a member of the opposite sex can therefore serve as a "defence mechanism" to diminish anxiety. Environmental factors, family systems, socialization, prenatal hormones, and the neuronal density of the hypothalamus may all be involved in gender identity disorders (Gale, 2001; Stonehouse, 2003; Zucker and Bradley, 1995, as cited in Moebius, 1998).

If we view sexual orientation as a continuum, then transsexuals vary in their positions along it. Sexual preference may vary for some individuals, whereas others may remain uncertain about their sexual orientation (Israel and Tarver, 1997). Some have always been aware of their gender identity and sexual orientation. For others, the discovery takes place after puberty.

Here is one (male-to-female) transsexual's reflection:

> I was verbal very early on, however, and even made up my own words to describe concepts that were beyond my vocabulary – and exploded in a rage when others didn't understand me. Like most autistic children, I had tantrums that would last for hours at a time.

> The origin of my gender issues is very hard to pinpoint. I knew for sure about age 13, when I first heard sex-change surgery was possible. As a child, if anyone had asked me, however, I would have said I was a boy, since that's what everyone told me I was. But I didn't particularly like the things boys did – my favourite toy when I was small was a talking boy doll, which my mother bought me over the objections of my grandmother.

> I didn't act on my gender issues until after I moved out at age 30. I tried to tell my parents and counsellors in my teens, but they chalked up the problems to the insecurity of adolescence, complicated by the cerebral palsy. It took a nervous breakdown and hospitalization for me to finally come to terms with what I was and begin transition.

> I quickly found out my life story didn't match those of other transsexuals. I am not hypersocial, for one, and women are expected in our society to be social creatures. I am also neither hyper-feminine nor extremely masculine, but somewhere in the middle, which seems to fit the profile of genetic AS females pretty well. It did lead to some self-doubt on my part – for a long time, I wondered if I made the right decision by transitioning. But I came to the conclusion after talking to AS women that if I had been born biologically female, I probably would have been much the same as I am now.

She adds:

> As to sexual preference, I was pretty much asexual – I didn't feel particularly attracted to either sex – until I started female hormones. Then I showed a definite attraction toward men. Thus, I didn't have my first sexual experience until I was about 37, after I had transitioned.

Manifestations of gender identity disorder can first be observed in children between the ages of two and four years. Parents frequently report their child's preference for opposite-sex clothing and toys (Gale, 2001).

Children and adolescents who explore gender roles may have many ensuing problems. The following deals with the assessment of a 13-year-old with AS.

> Manuel's parents were worried about his behaviour. He had been acting like a girl for about one year. He wore dresses and lipstick at home and claimed to be pregnant. His parents forbade this behaviour at school and during any outings. They were concerned about their son and the impact of these behaviours on his social relationships. He had no close friends at school and preferred to spend time alone. He play-acted (singing, dancing, dressing up) on weekends and performed for his parents and his older sister's friends.
>
> At our first contact, Manuel was shy and avoided looking at me. He didn't understand why he had to talk to me about himself. According to him, it was quite obvious that he was a girl. After having talked about his interests, the music that he listened to, and the things that he did with his sister and her friends, he seemed more open to talking about his imaginary "pregnancy". He lifted his sweater and showed me his (flat) stomach and stated that he carried a baby. At first, his statements might have appeared psychotic (individuals with AS were, for years, diagnosed as psychotic or schizophrenic due to their odd words and gestures, especially when taken out of context) but, in this case, Manuel simply had a rich imagination.
>
> During the second session we drew pictures of boys and girls (doing activities that they enjoy) and I asked him which drawing most represented him. He quickly pointed to the boy. He then pointed to the girl and stated that she looked like me. When I asked him which he preferred, he pointed to the girl. Later on, he came close to me to see if I was wearing nail polish. He drew my attention to the nail polish that he wore on his toes. He told me that girls were beautiful (especially blondes!) and that he was in love with a girl at school and he wished that she loved him in return. At the end of the session he imitated his favourite musical band by singing and dancing. His mother confirmed that he identified with the lead singer (who was male) but he interjected and reminded me that he was a girl. This gender alternation allowed us to explore the characteristics of boys and girls. Manuel appreciated boys but preferred the presence of girls. With respect to other symptoms, he didn't show any signs of anxiety or depression. He was isolated, but didn't complain because his imagination was filled with people and friends. I proposed that he complete the Gender Identity Profile (Israel and Tarver, 1997) to explore his identification, sexual attraction, and behaviour. At that time, the results did not indicate an identity conflict; Manuel was exploring and playing with both genders, a common behaviour of prepubescent children. Identity usually becomes fixed during puberty. I recommended that Manuel go to therapy in order to manage his behaviour and offer him support.

The Gender Identity Profile (Israel and Tarver, 1997) consists of 40 items on imagination, behaviour, transvestism, sexual conduct, steps taken (hormone replacement therapy, electrolysis, surgery, etc.), desires, and psychological symptoms (depression, anxiety, etc.). In a complementary document, Dr Israel added a series of questions pertaining to individuals with autism (Israel, personal communication). She is interested in the relationship between autism and gender identity conflicts and recommends that therapy should be available for transsexuals with AS.

Rosenberg (2002) recommends treatments based on encouraging self-acceptance and educating over those that try to change individuals' sexual identification. Better results are noted when therapy works on consolidating self-esteem and acceptance. Israel and Tarver (1997) suggest the use of tools such as questionnaires, letters, or other resources that help the person along in their steps towards surgical transition.

So far, few studies have investigated the link between autism, AS and transsexualism or gender identity disorder. Mukkades (2002) cites four empirical studies on gender identity, transsexualism, and autism. Of these, Abelson (1981) was the first to assess gender identity development in an autistic child. Williams, Allard and Lonnie (1996), Landen and Rasmussen (1997) and Mukkades (2002) investigated transvestic behaviour and found unusual preoccupations, fantasies, obsessive-compulsive behaviours, socioaffective developmental difficulties, and attachments to "feminine objects". In fact, Landen and Rasmussen (1997) suggested a possible comorbidity between autism and transsexualism. Lately Gallucci, Hackerman, and Schmidt (2005) discuss a case of gender identity disorder in a man with AS, and clinical studies have found a 7:1 male to female ratio for gender identity disorder (Bradley and Zucker, 1997). Cohen-Kettenis (2003) conducted a study with 488 children between the ages of 3 and 13 years who were referred to the Child and Adolescent Gender Identity Clinic in Toronto (Canada) and the Gender Clinic in Utrecht (Netherlands). Boys were found to have less overall social competency and inferior peer relations – characteristics also found in AS. However, Cohen-Kettenis did not establish a relationship between the two conditions.

The possible link between AS and gender identity disorder has given rise to several interesting debates. Some view the issue as one involving a continuum of difference. One woman with AS in Cohen-Kettenis' (2003) study revealed that she was aware of her difference from an early age. Her sexuality followed along the same continuum of diversity; she didn't feel that the two conditions were independent of one another. Another participant asserted that autism or AS was a manifestation of her gender conflict. Some individuals received childhood diagnoses of "neurosis due to opposite-sex identification", "psychosis involving delusions in gender identification", "asocialization and transvestism", "non-specified autism and gender identity disorder", and "schizophrenia and castration anxiety". Dual diagnoses must be considered for certain individuals with AS.

In interviews, adults with autism, Pervasive Developmental Disorder (PDD), and AS said of their understanding of this dual condition:

> If a girl acts and dresses in a particular way, I should be a girl in a boy's body. There's a difference between acting like a girl and wanting to become a girl.

> My identity disorder first had to do with my body. My conflict didn't involve the social implications of acting and being like a girl, but of having the wrong body.

> I have always been annoyed by gender expectations. I am annoyed that there is a DSM entry for gender identity disorder. Identity is a cultural phenomenon. I am annoyed that science attempts to treat cultural problems with the same tools as they treat cancers. I believe autism to be a cultural problem. If autism was treated as a set of personality traits, temperament and the like (stuff we use in professional development courses), I believe our contribution to the world could be significant and unique.

> One of the real dangers I see is if young people are forced to fit societal expectations without the opportunity and tools to discover themselves. This happened to me, and I'm still going through the process of self-discovery, and dealing with "re-emerging traits". Fortunately, my memory tends to be a bit of a "log file", and little details (emotions, etc.) that were overlooked at the time are still preserved.

Some individuals experience autistic spectrum disorders (including PDD and AS) first, and the gender identity conflict emerges later. This makes sense in that gender identity is crystallized during puberty, whereas symptoms of autism and PDDs are observed in children aged three or four years. Although gender identity conflicts are reported in young children (aged between three and seven), very few studies have been conducted on this sample. Data are mainly obtained through clinical observation. While genitals and body hair are concrete and practical manifestations of gender in younger individuals with AS, manifestations of gender identity in adults are much more complex.

Martine Stonehouse, a transsexual woman with AS, has written an autobiography entitled *Stilted Rainbow: The Story of My Life on the Autistic Spectrum and a Gender Identity Conflict* (2002). She was referred for social and psychiatric assessment when she was seven years old. Martine showed "a poor self-image and confused identity" from childhood. Her psychiatrist also mentioned castration anxiety and effeminate behaviour. Since then she has fought for the rights of transsexuals, is a member of discussion groups for transsexuals with PDDs, and has been cited in a variety of newspapers and magazines (*The Toronto Star, XTRA Magazine*). The following extract is taken from her book.

> Another thing happened to come along and caused a great upheaval in my life, it was called puberty. I could sense that something was very wrong and I

wasn't developing as I thought I should. Up until this point I didn't relate myself to a gender, I was just myself. If anything I related and felt more towards girls and women, but I didn't actively pursue it. Now my body was being forced into a gender, and not what I thought it would be.

Like most changes, I did not take well to it. Girls' bodies were developing differently than mine, and I didn't know why. I began to feel alienated and confused with myself, I had many questions but no one to turn to for help. As I began to develop, I began to grow hair on my face and all over my body. This made me feel like a gorilla or the wolfman. My voice remained high and I did develop small breasts, but I wasn't like the other girls. I felt betrayed as I began to turn into a man. It was like turning into the monster in the horror movies.

Back at school some of the girls in the class would tease me in suggestive ways, which I felt uncomfortable about. I was attracted to some of them, but I also envied them and felt shut out from their world, even though I felt the same as them. I never dated during my high school years and basically I have not had any intimate relationships in my life.

I managed to cope through all this by becoming extremely focused in my hobby of collecting license plates, people were not important to me at this point in my life, focusing on my hobbies was safer than dealing with the world.

In June 1994, I transitioned from my "male" self to my new identity as a woman. I now feel much more comfortable with myself and I have never looked back. There was one thing that remained unresolved in my life, but I didn't know that it was at that point in my life.

A chance comment by my supervisor "I can't teach you common sense; you either have it or you don't," sent me on a quest to unlock the mysteries of my childhood. At first I thought I might have Attention Deficit Hyperactivity Disorder, but in seeing a specialist, we soon found out there was more. It seemed I had an Autism Spectrum Disorder, known as Asperger's Syndrome.

Martine has also written a collection of poetry (forthcoming). Here is one of her poems:

An Autistic Android

I live on a world, so alien to me, How did I get here? Why am I so
    different?
Wanting to be like the rest of you, But not knowing how to fit in with
    your world.
Your ways and manners are strange to me, And trying to decipher your
    customs,
Seems like an undertaking in vain.
Like a scientist from a different world, I watch and observe to learn how
    to act,
So that I can imitate your behavior, And attempt to fit in with your kind.

But it's your feelings and emotions, I just cannot grasp.
For I'm an Autistic Android, That is not programmed for these feelings,
My world is of logic and facts, Not understanding how you relate.
I long to feel the things you express, The joy you feel, the laughter you laugh,
Understanding what love is, To let one's self go,
And experience a world without logic. I guess it is just not to be,
For these feelings do not seem to be in me.
Maybe, someday I will find another android like me, a companion who I can understand,
And one who will understand me.
For a relationship with an earthling, certainly does not seem possible,
As their relationships confuse me, just as I confuse them.
There must be other androids like me, from our far away planet called Autism.
It gets lonely on this world called Earth, when its people are so foreign to me.
So, I search this planet constantly, looking for others like me,
To join me in research, as we probe this planet together, relating our findings to each other,
and understanding our logic together.
I'm sending a message to all Auties out there, hoping for a companion to share.
To help each other through this world so alien to us, knowing that we understand each other,
And reassuring for us, that someone out there really does care.
Is there someone out there?

Sexual diversity and gender identity are important for people with AS. Psychological symptoms associated with lack of comprehension and peer and family reactions only add to the difficulties they experience. If we take a pathological perspective on gender identity or sexual orientation, we will only push these individuals along the path towards delinquency and abnormality and limit any dialogue they may have with health professionals.

Further studies need to be conducted in this area in order to obtain a better understanding of the factors involved in the development of gender identity and to provide relevant treatments to meet the needs of individuals struggling with gender identity conflict.

Chapter 5

Couples, intimacy, and sexuality

This chapter explores the sexual and intimate relationships of couples affected by AS: in other words, where one or both partners have AS. We will explore issues related to those adjustments that may be required of a partner with AS and of a neurotypical partner in a relationship, and will also examine relationships where both partners have AS. In a couple, the expression of traits and behaviours linked to AS vary according to several factors, such as prior experiences, self-disclosure, acceptance of the syndrome, quality of communication, family situation, mutual support, and the partner's motivation. This chapter discusses relationship factors such as intimacy, empathy, sexual desire, commitment, and couple therapy. It concludes with thoughts on couples and sexuality expressed by an individual with AS.

Intimacy

The main component of couple relationships – intimacy – is difficult to define. The Latin word *intimus* refers to what is most interior (Dubé, 1994). "Intimacy" has been defined as a need for sharing and affection (McAdams, 1988; Weiss, 1973). If this need is satisfied, the individual is reassured about their self-worth, and this improves their social integration. Erickson (1963) stressed that being in an intimate relationship with someone else involves making sacrifices and compromises in order to maintain commitment. Hatfield (1984) adds that intimacy is the process in which two individuals try to get closer to one another in order to know each other at the deepest level. Personal goals, wishes and dreams tend to be fulfilled in intimate relationships.

All individuals have their own ideas as to what constitutes intimacy and every couple has its own experiences. For some, intimacy is represented by walking hand in hand, sharing emotions, having a meal together, or having a loving or sexual exchange. Intimacy can be a vague concept for many individuals with AS. It isn't that they don't have the desire to be intimate with a partner; rather, many are limited in their experience of interpersonal relationships. Lack of intimacy is a major source of unhappiness for couples affected by AS. Sexual satisfaction (in terms of sexual frequency and quality) is not necessarily an indication that a couple is happy and fulfilled. However, some neurotypical partners report that their counterparts with AS assume that a satisfying relationship means having an active sexual life. Sexuality is an important component of intimacy, but it is not the only one. The interpretation of intimacy in terms of the physical or tangible is not uncommon among those with the Asperger profile.

Sexual desire

Sexual desire, the longing for closeness with someone, is also a component of intimacy. Sexual desire can manifest itself in many ways. It can be expressed behaviourally (through physical closeness, sexual caresses, etc.) and emotionally (through affection, sharing feelings, etc.). Low sexual desire is the most common complaint of individuals and/or couples seen for sexual and couple problems. Several factors are related to low sexual desire, and it is important to assess if a change in the level of a person's desire is temporary or more permanent. Stress, overwork, anxiety, or destabilizing situations can sometimes explain short-term changes in the level of desire.

If a couple has been experiencing low sexual desire for some time and the temporary changes mentioned above are not the cause, four areas should be explored:

- There may be a decrease in the frequency of sexual activity. It is important to assess the discrepancy between *actual* and *desired* levels of sexual frequency. In general, men and women have different perceptions of sexual frequency. Men tend to overestimate the number of actual sexual contacts while women tend to underestimate them. This tendency is rarely observed in couples where one or both partners have AS. On the contrary, partners with AS report precise and exact frequencies, although in a few cases, the partner with AS may seem "amnesic" in this respect. In general, individuals with AS seem to be more satisfied with a low frequency of sexual activity than the general population (Hénault *et al.*, 2003). A lack of prior sexual experience among individuals with AS and the fact that a lower proportion of them are in a relationship may explain this difference.

- Avoidance behaviours, including making excuses, going to bed before or after the partner, generally conveying a lack of desire, or any other rituals that elude sexual contact are also related to low sexual desire. Such an avoidance routine, once set, can be difficult to modify, while circumscribed interests may also become an "excuse" to avoid intimacy with their partner.

- The third area involves couples' sexual repertoires. Exploration and novelty are important ingredients for maintaining or increasing sexual desire, but individuals with AS prefer routines and repetitive sequences of behaviour. When the sexual script is rigid, limited, and predictable, arousal levels tend to decrease and sex becomes unfulfilling in the long term.

- A lack of emotional communication about affection, intimacy, and sexuality can have a negative impact on sexual desire. Sex can become a taboo subject, which further leads to a decrease in affectionate behaviours and the development of negative thoughts. Emotional communication goes above and beyond routine superficial exchange. It involves sharing emotions and intimate thoughts. Such exchanges should be frequent to help build complicity between partners. Partners with AS may have difficulty with intimate exchanges. They may be quite uncomfortable with intimate communication since it is so different from their usual logical, tangible style. This can be accompanied by a reduction in time spent on activities as a couple. "Quality" time spent together is important and involves couples coming together to share and consolidate their intimacy. Examples of less-than-optimal exchanges include partners having a discussion while engaging in household chores, one partner making a telephone call to the other between two appointments, verbal exchanges with partners being in separate rooms, one partner summarizing the day at meal time, a partner starting a discussion at bedtime. While these examples can lead to rich and interesting conversations, the major problem with them is their lack of affectionate exchange and intimacy, especially when these are the only times when a couple connects. When even these moments are isolated from one another and large time spans (several days or weeks) go by before the discussion is taken up again, it becomes much more difficult to establish an intimate affectionate relationship with your partner.

A man with AS didn't realize the importance of intimate moments. His partner suffered from their lack of intimate exchanges and affection. When she articulated this, he took the comment as a criticism and found refuge in his favourite activity, which caused the distance between them to be maintained. Another couple expressed how dissatisfied they were about their numerous fights. The partner with AS expressed his attraction to and desire for his partner solely through sexual exchanges. Despite their varied and frequent sexual life the neurotypical partner was deeply concerned with the lack of connection between the purely "sexual" and the missing "emotional" dimensions of their relationship. Her partner explained that sexuality was the concrete proof of his desire for her. Sexual needs were met here, but intimacy needs were not.

This dynamic is quite common in couples where one partner has AS. The dynamic can be similar or totally different when two partners with AS are involved. If they share the same perspective, they will adjust to each other quite easily. If their perspectives diverge, the couple will be more likely to encounter difficulties. Is it possible to maintain desire by fostering intimacy? Partners must understand that this is an active process where shared responsibility is required. Blaming each other will only contribute to the vicious cycle of avoidance and anger.

Affective communication

Establishing good communication is the first step leading to mutual understanding. However, couples need to agree on what constitutes intimacy. It is virtually impossible to address the issue of low sexual desire without first looking at the components of intimacy. One useful exercise involves establishing each partner's definition of intimacy. Each partner lists all the words and activities that he or she feels represent intimacy. There are no right or wrong answers here. By comparing the lists, partners can discuss the similarities and differences, and what they each feel constitutes intimacy. If one partner's list is limited, the discussion can help them develop it. The exercise should *never* be confrontational. The goal is to have a common dialogue and a constructive exchange. Partners can then choose to work on one element on the lists per week until they are satisfied with their level of intimacy. The rigidity experienced by individuals with AS is often due to their failure to understand their partner's desires and a tendency to be egocentric. Sharing, compromise, and sensitivity are essential to a harmonious relationship with a partner.

The communication exercises discussed in Chapter 3, especially the importance of speaking in "I" messages, can be useful to help discuss the notion of "quality time". A journal can be completed on a weekly basis to record progress and can include some of the elements listed in Box 5.1 (p.94).

Waiting for one partner to take the initiative can lead to laziness on one side and frustration on the other. Furthermore, if only one partner is responsible for gestures of attention and affection, they may feel taken for granted. The greater the number of physical and relationship obstacles, the more difficult it will be to experience intimacy.

Box 5.1: Couple homework

Week: _____

1. Provide an example of good, positive communication within your relationship.

_____
_____
_____
_____
_____
_____

2. What intimate moments have taken place over the past week (shared activities, sexual contact, etc.)?

_____
_____
_____
_____
_____
_____

3. Describe a misunderstanding that you discussed and solved between yourselves.

_____
_____
_____
_____
_____
_____

4. Rate how successful you think the following aspects of your relationship have been this week on a scale of 1 (not at all successful) to 10 (very successful):

a. Communication: c. Sexuality:

b. Intimacy: d. Daily activities:

Couple dynamics

Expressing commitment, confidence, and affection requires interpersonal skills (L'Abate and Sloan, 1984; Margolin, 1982), but three further elements are necessary to establish intimacy between two people:

1. The sharing of ideas, beliefs, and dreams.

2. Sexuality and affection.

3. The recognition of one's own value and individual needs.

Ron Hedgcock (2002), an adult with AS, gives an insight into how AS has affected his relationships in this respect:

> I was very slow in the development of sexual knowledge or the comprehension of my own sexuality. With no instinct for self-protection, I was frequently bullied or abused by the other kids. I found that others rarely included me. A select grouping of friends developed in my life…very few males, but quite a lot of women, who tended to regard me far more like a brother or even a girlfriend, than as a potential mate. Quite heterosexual, but I experienced none of the proverbial sexual chemistry with anyone. I always took it for granted that I would marry and have children, just as in the family I had grown up in. But I never understood Love or Intimacy or bonding in the terms they carry in the world outside. "Reading" or "mind-reading" other people had never been part of my experience. Love and marriage appeared to me to be pragmatic and simple. I had never been conscious of my parents having to "work" at their marriage; and I had no conception that marriage could be a difficult or dangerous business. The very choice of a partner was a simple business to me – based purely on a pragmatic "liking" for each other and some mutual interests. Sex was simply something that just happened enjoyably and easily between the friendly partners. No subtle or underlying condition was required.
>
> Well, it must be said that a series of marriages happened for me. They left me (and doubtless the poor ladies too) utterly bewildered. Life with another person appeared to me to be chaotic. While I could satisfactorily get on with others in the outside world, intimate living with another left me uncomfortable and stressed. Quite clearly, my lack of "connection" to my wives ruined the marriages. No-one knew anything of Asperger's Syndrome, and the essential question about me and my inability to love or to be intimate, was virtually, "Am I mad, bad or just disgustingly thoughtless?"
>
> The person you "love" is, still everyday after 20–30 years together, a puzzle, a new thing to be considered, and even a hurdle to overcome. You never know them – you never had the thrill of "chemistry" with them, or anyone else. Every interaction with them is an unknown. You never have "gut" feelings about them…no instinct that gives warning or approval. Nothing in body, mind or spirit is transformed or motivated by "love". Love, intimacy and bonding, are mysteries. Sex and Love are tucked into compartments in your life.

Several books have been written on the experiences of couples living with AS. *The Other Half of Asperger Syndrome* (Aston, 2001), *Aspergers in Love* (Aston, 2003), *Asperger Syndrome and Adults… Is Anyone Listening?* (Rodman, 2003), *An Asperger Marriage* (Slater-Walker and Slater-Walker, 2002), and *Asperger Syndrome and Long-Term Relationships* (Stanford, 2002) are interesting references for couples. Couple dynamics have to be addressed by considering the partner with AS since it is this condition that affects the dynamics of a couple's relationship on a daily basis. Rigidity, circumscribed interests, and rituals can lead the partner with AS to make unusual or excessive demands. The other partner will have to adjust to this since these characteristics are inherent in AS. Recognizing and accepting the diagnosis of AS is of primary importance in the relationship. Denial by either the individual himself or his partner will only lead to incomprehension and resistance to change. Blaming the person with AS or making them responsible for the couple's difficulties will only serve to provoke defensive attitudes and behaviours. Communication and intimacy will suffer greatly.

However, couples do not need to struggle with these problems alone. Attwood (2003b) has proposed 11 strategies to help strengthen couple relationships which include recognizing the diagnosis and being motivated to learn, relationship counselling, improving mutual understanding, occasional "holidays" from one's partner, learning to manage emotions and communicating openly and effectively. Obtaining external sources of support (support groups such as *www.FAAAS.org*, therapy, family support, local groups, etc.) also helps re-establish balance. The couple should engage in social activities together and individually.

Some couples who come to therapy report a routine and unsatisfactory sexual life. Others express satisfaction with their sexual life, but note an absence of emotional exchange in the relationship. Each couple's story is unique. However, some particularities are observed in terms of sexual intimacy, as we have discussed, and also in terms of the perceived lack of empathy of partners with AS.

Empathy

The total or partial absence of empathy involves a general feeling of indifference towards the well-being or happiness of others. AS itself, depression, grief, or partner dissatisfaction can all affect the person with AS. Providing emotional and physical support is not part of the AS mind-set, and this may create the impression that someone with AS doesn't care for others. Difficulties related to decoding and managing emotions and the theory of mind are in part responsible for this apparent lack of empathy among some partners with AS. In some cases, a form of narcissism can aggravate this lack of empathy; individuals become pre-occupied with their own needs and things that concern them directly. Totally absorbed by their circumscribed interests, individuals with AS tend to ignore external sources of stimulation, such as others' feelings.

Logical and literal thinking can also be problematic in emotional contexts. When a partner makes an announcement about something emotional, such as a serious illness, the death of a family member, or losing their job, the news may be received dispassionately by people with AS ("it's not serious, go see a doctor", "such is life", "it wasn't the right job for you", "you're making a big deal out of it", "so what?"), giving the impression that they are insensitive to what their partners are experiencing. This can lead to conflict.

Empathy is an important part of mental health (Foreman, 2003). Robert W. Levenson (cited in Foreman, 2003) discusses three forms of empathy: cognitive, emotional, and compassionate. Cognitive empathy is the capacity to "know" what another person feels without feeling any kindness or emotion for the other. Emotional empathy refers to "feeling what someone [else] is feeling", and compassion is to do something in response to another's emotional experience (e.g. offer a hug). Andrew Meltzoff (cited in Foreman, 2003) argues that "empathy, including the sophisticated talent for treating others like as you would like to be treated, builds on primitive imitation".

However, while the ability to imitate facial expressions develops from an early age in neurotypical individuals, it remains deficient in people with AS. Interventions based on recognizing and managing emotions can therefore be very useful for helping an individual with AS develop empathy. It is helpful to do this in the presence of the neurotypical partner to build understanding.

Sexual intimacy

Therapy can be useful for enhancing sexual intimacy, changing behaviours, and modifying sexual scripts (routines related to sexual activities). Sexuality meets various needs in a relationship, including physical and emotional closeness, pleasure, fantasy, duty, and routine. The needs and expectations of both partners are not always the same. Problems can arise when each of the partners has a totally different concept of sexuality. Thought-provoking and explorative exercises can help increase sexual intimacy. Below are some activities that are frequently suggested in the context of couple therapy.

The first exercise involves exploring erogenous zones, the most sensitive parts of the body. Sexual, sensual, or tactile pleasure can be experienced when erogenous zones are caressed. Partners are presented with a sheet of paper showing two bodies (the couple). Each partner must circle what they believe to be the other's erogenous zones and rate the intensity of the pleasure experienced by the other when these areas are caressed. Ratings range from one to ten. A score of 1 corresponds to very little pleasure, 5 represents moderate pleasure, and 10 intense pleasure. The goal of this exercise is to compare partners' perceptions. Despite its apparent simplicity, the exercise addresses several issues.

In general, partners have a tendency to project their own preferences and over-evaluate others' sensitive body parts. The exercise can also reveal a lack of knowledge of the other's body. For example, a partner who appreciates genital caresses circles the genital area of their partner and indicates a high pleasure rating of 9. When questioned, the other partner reports that they appreciate genital caresses, but give them the lesser rating of 6; instead, they report preferring caresses to the upper body, namely to the chest and neck. Similarly, they will circle the upper body parts of the other and provide high sensitivity ratings for those.

Many partners and couples tend to limit their exploration to sexual body parts. The exercise here is therefore much more global. Couples must take the time to explore the entirety of the body, from head to toe. Caresses that are only directed to the genitals can of course give pleasure, but they may sometimes be perceived as invasive.

After completing this exercise, the couple should be encouraged to discuss foreplay. Couples often bypass foreplay in favour of sexual intercourse, and yet foreplay serves to increase desire and arousal. Caresses, kisses, hugs, and affectionate behaviours cause the muscles of the internal genitalia, more specifically the pubococcygian muscle, to relax. The relaxed state helps individuals focus on pleasant sensations that accompany lovemaking and put aside their preoccupations. Some individuals with AS deal with foreplay in a mechanical manner and don't let themselves experience the moment and savour the pleasure that accompanies the caresses. Their partners can therefore feel as if they don't really exist or are being reduced to a sexual object.

The tactile sensitivities of partners with AS must also be considered. One adult with AS reports:

> I find it very difficult to give or receive intimate caresses. So much emotional and physical information is transmitted at the same time. I feel overwhelmed and my body shuts down. I feel panicky, I tremble, and I try to get myself out of the situation. If my partner is gentle and patient, I can relax and trust him. I can then experience touch and caresses quite differently and I can achieve pleasure.

It is possible for people with AS who have tactile sensitivities to become more comfortable with intimate touch. Their partner's patience, tenderness, and trust are crucial elements. Both partners must have good communication skills so that they can share their experiences. The exercise above and the exercise on sensate focus below, can help couples learn how to touch one another in pleasurable ways that are respectful of tactile sensitivities, and they also help them to discover the body parts that give rise to sexual/sensual pleasure. Each individual is unique and reactions may vary, but these exercises aim to decrease apprehension, anxiety, and aversive reactions.

COUPLES, INTIMACY, AND SEXUALITY

The following exercise on sensate focus, targets a couple's sexual script. It is highly likely that, due to the nature of AS, sexual activities are quite routine in terms of their frequency, foreplay, positions, and so on, as discussed earlier in this chapter. The aim is to develop more spontaneity and explore the variety of sexual contacts that can take place between partners. Sensate focus was developed by Masters and Johnson (1970) and has been adapted in various ways (Jacobson and Gurman, 1995; Keesling, 1993; Paradis and Lafond, 1990). Box 5.2 (p.100) describes the steps of sensate focus. This exercise should be accompanied by discussions around consent and about the experience.

Sensate focus is important for couples affected by AS in that it allows them to go beyond the caresses that automatically lead to penetration. Exploring a partner's body, feeling pleasure, and taking the time to experience the activity lead to changes in routine and allow new behaviours to be integrated into the couple's sexual script. This process involves openness on the part of couples. Motivation is also required, for it is much more difficult to change habits than it is to reproduce the same routines over and over again. The sexual life of couples will be enriched and sexual desire will improve.

Individual interventions may also be necessary with some partners. Lonnie Barbach's *Loving Together: Sexual Enrichment Program* (1997) consists of thought-provoking and practical exercises that take place over an intensive ten-week period. The activities that make up this programme can easily be integrated into a more elaborate therapeutic process.

Foreplay and sexual positions can be discussed using pictures and photographs. Behavioural sequences can be analysed in such a way as to expand on a couple's pre-existing sexual scripts. The aim is for the couple to try to avoid overly rigid routines during sexual relations. Partners appreciate constructing sequences of behaviour that meet their needs. Talking about foreplay (using images and educational videos) can also teach partners about the various types of caresses. This can be particularly useful for individuals with AS given their often limited sexual experience.

The most important ingredient in all of these exercises is the partners' commitment. Engaging in a therapeutic process reflects their need to share and evolve as a couple. Both partners must be motivated because the process requires time and energy. Therapy extends beyond weekly sessions; homework exercises must be completed during the week. Changes are sometimes painful, especially for partners with AS who are accustomed to their routines. They need to learn to consider their partners' requests and desires. Assertiveness and positive communication are important throughout the process. Sex therapy must be adapted to the needs and experiences of individuals with AS and should involve all aspects of sexuality. Despite being laborious, sex therapy is a worthwhile investment for couples.

Box 5.2: Sensate focus

The purpose of this exercise is to experience intimate and sensual discovery without engaging in penetration. You should explore the sensations associated with pleasure and share them with your partner.

Try to prepare for the moment by creating a relaxing and pleasant environment. Make sure that you will not be disturbed for the next 30 to 60 minutes. You can dim the lights, listen to music, take a bath or a shower with your partner, get comfortable... You can experience each step in a different place or establish a different ambience.

Step 1

During this first step, each of you (one after another or both at the same time) will take time to explore your partner's body with your hands and/or mouth. Start with caresses that you are comfortable with. If some gestures bother you (or your partner), don't continue them. Each of you should focus your attention on the pleasant or unpleasant sensations that you receive.

Let your partner know what caresses are pleasant, unpleasant, or painful.

It is important to place the emphasis on non-genital body parts. Therefore do not touch your partner's genitals, anus, or breasts. The objective is to progressively explore your partner's body (from head to toe) without there necessarily being any sexual arousal.

At the end of the experience, communicate about what you got out of the exercise; share your experiences.

Step 2

Follow the same guidelines as for Step 1, but you may now caress your partner's whole body, including genitals, anus, and breasts. If you are not comfortable with some body parts, avoid them. The goal of this step is to discover bodily sensations. Rhythmic stimulation (of a masturbatory type) is not recommended because it could lead to orgasm, which is not the goal of exploration.

You can do this second step one after the other or simultaneously. After the exercise, you should also share what you felt as you were giving and receiving the caresses.

Step 3

You can now caress your partner manually or orally until he/she reaches orgasm. Vaginal penetration is not recommended. The goal is for you to experiment with new caresses and sexual behaviours. You can take turns to do this, one after another, or do this simultaneously.

It is useful to talk about this exercise at the end of this third step. You should each express what you appreciated and what positive elements came out of exploring your partner's body. The goal is to broaden your repertoire of sexual activities as a couple.

Adapted from Masters and Johnson (1970)

Chapter 6

The sociosexual education programme

Sexual education programmes

According to Family Planning Queensland (2001) and the National Information Center for Children and Youth with Disabilities (1992), sexual education programmes should provide information, develop values, encourage interpersonal skills, and help individuals learn to be responsible in their sexual behaviour. Programmes should consider sexuality in its entirety and include concepts of intimacy, desire, communication, love, deviance, and satisfaction (Griffiths *et al.*, 2002; Haracopos and Pedersen, 1999). They should also discuss sexual and gender identity, sexual needs, and sexual development.

As suggested in the literature (Chipouras *et al.*, 1982; Griffiths *et al.*, 1989; Hellemans, 1996), a structured sexual education programme designed to meet the needs of the Asperger population should be part of the services offered and extended to individuals with AS. The National Information Center for Children and Youth with Disabilities (1992), Kempton (1993), and Hingsburger (1993), all state that the more individuals with autism and AS are informed about sexuality, the better they are able to make informed and autonomous choices. This not only decreases their risk of experiencing sexual abuse, it also allows them access to a rewarding social and sexual life.

Several authors have recognized the need for sexual education for individuals with autism (e.g. Attwood, personal communication; Gray *et al.*, 1996; Haracopos and Pedersen, 1999; Hellemans, 1996; Hingsburger, 1993). This has yet to be extended to the Asperger population. Sexual education programmes do exist for individuals with intellectual disabilities (e.g. Kaeser and O'Neill, 1987), but few address the specific needs of those with high functioning autism or AS. One preliminary version of such a programme has been proposed by Haracopos and Pedersen (1999), and Kempton (1993), a pioneer in specialized sexual education, has published a sociosexual education programme designed for individuals with a PDD. This programme provides excellent information on social skills and interpersonal relationships, but topics related to sexuality are limited and the educational material is not sufficiently practical. Other social skills programmes (e.g. Ouellet and L'Abbé, 1986; Soyner and Desnoyers Hurley, 1990) also provide good information on socialization, but only briefly address the notions of sexuality and intimacy. The *SexoTrousse* (Lemay, 1996), *Programme d'éducation à la vie affective, amoureuse et sexuelle* (Desaulniers, 2001), and the *Life Horizons I and II* (Kempton, 1999) programmes, developed for people with intellectual disabilities and PDD, have the advantage of including practical material and pertinent activities, but they are not adapted to the needs of individuals with AS.

The *Programme d'éducation sexuelle* (Durocher and Fortier, 1999) appears to be the most promising programme for young people with AS, given their sexual and cognitive profile. The activities in it are practical and full of imagery, and require high levels of participation. The programme was designed to be administered to groups and focuses on interpersonal exchanges and social contacts. It has been used to help individuals with a variety of behavioural disorders such as aggression, opposition, and hyperactivity. This programme forms the foundation for the sociosexual education programme for individuals with AS presented in this book.

This programme is divided into 12 workshops related to sexuality, which have been developed specifically to meet the needs of the Asperger population. Developed from Durocher and Fortier's (1999) programme, more practical activities have been included, visual support has been increased, and there is more repetition of exercises so as to allow participants to understand the material better. Various other resources such as videos, Internet sites and assessment sheets are also suggested, including the *Gaining Face* software (Team Asperger, 2000); the *Mind-Reading* software (Baron Cohen *et al.*, 2004); pictures from the *SexoTrousse* (Lemay, 1996); cognitive behaviour strategies, etc. The topics that are addressed in the 12 workshops of the programme include:

- love and friendship
- physiological aspects
- sexual intercourse and other behaviours
- emotions
- STDs, HIV, and prevention of unwanted pregnancy
- sexual orientation
- alcohol and drugs
- sexual abuse and inappropriate behaviours
- sexism and violence in romantic relationships
- management of emotions, theory of mind, and intimacy.

These workshops address the sexual reality of individuals with AS, as defined by Haracopos and Pedersen (1999) and Kempton (1993). Techniques such as role-playing, rehearsal, and group sessions are used. In order to facilitate these interventions, each workshop is accompanied by notes for the group leader. The modifications to Durocher and Fortier's programme have made it possible to offer an innovative programme to adolescents and adults with AS. It can be offered to individuals, but the section on social skills would need to be modified in that case since the activities were designed to be administered to a group. Although previously unpublished, this programme has been empirically validated and tested in practice with four groups (Hénault *et al.*, 2003).

The structure of the sociosexual education programme for individuals with Asperger's Syndrome

The sociosexual programme that we used and present in this book consists of 12 workshops. Each workshop includes a support sheet for the group leader, the required materials, and all instructions. The activities in the workshops can be adapted depending on the group (according to age, special needs, receptivity, etc.). In general, participants should be divided into groups according to their ages (from 16 to 20 years, 20 to 30 years, 30 to 40 years, etc.). Whenever possible, it is always preferable to include both genders in a group. Boys are always curious to hear what girls think and vice versa. Each workshop was developed to last about 90 minutes; however, a group leader could easily decide to divide it into two 45-minute workshops. The 12-session formula described in this book can certainly be modified. Activities and exercises can be repeated and the programme can be extended to over 20 workshops or more. However, the results (borrowed from Hénault *et al.*, 2003) described here are for the 12-session, 90-minute format.

How the sociosexual education programme helps individuals with Asperger's Syndrome

When used with the four groups previously mentioned, this programme offered significant help in terms of intervention and sexual education for participants with high functioning autism and AS. The collaboration, respect, and interest shown by the participants indicated their motivation to participate in the programme. The subject of sexuality itself evoked much curiosity, because a programme on this topic was new to most of them. The intervention programme responded to and met a specific need.

In light of the nature of the intervention and the topics addressed, personal questions and disclosures on the part of the participants were to be expected. Each workshop was followed by a 30-minute period in which participants were invited to discuss any concerns. After a session in which we had discussed sexual behaviours and preferences, an adolescent with fetishistic tendencies asked to talk confidentially about the subject. Similarly, following the workshop on sexual abuse, another adolescent revealed in confidence the inappropriate behaviours of one of his family members. The "Information for the group leader" offer suggestions on how to address a variety of difficult issues like these that could come up after to a meeting. In this way it is possible to foster the individual's expression of healthy sexuality in parallel with group activities, without compromising confidentiality.

The programme's format is another of its significant strengths. Because the intervention takes place over 12 consecutive weeks, participants are able to develop friendships while interacting with one another. Group activities make it easier for group members to become close because they require members to socialize with each other. As the quality of interpersonal relationships within the group improves, friendship develops. During the last two workshops we observed this happening among the participants. Two participants discovered that they shared a common passion for wrestling. They exchanged magazines and began meeting one another outside of the group context. In another group, three participants engaged in activities together on a weekly basis. One participant introduced her favourite activity, bowling, to the group. Two adults in one group found that they had a passion for computers in common and an adolescent in another group introduced someone else to drawing. Developments like these were observed in all four of the groups.

Participating in a group also helps individuals to reduce any self-centred narcissistic attitudes they may have. Social skills enable them to become more open to the experiences of others, helping to reduce attitudes such as "I know everything" or "Everyone is ignorant", which were observed in some individuals in the programme. The reactions of their peers to these and inappropriate attitudes or behaviours are very useful during the workshops. For example, after they had watched a video on sexual abuse, some participants commented on the inappropriateness and detrimental effects of the behaviour they had seen on both victims and perpetrators, and these comments had an effect on those who tended more towards sexual aggression. Similarly, a discussion and a short video on masturbation helped an adolescent with high functioning autism to make changes to his inappropriate behaviour, which his mother later confirmed. The improved behaviour was still being maintained at the last follow-up three months after the programme had ended.

The use of stimulating visual materials in the workshops (videos, photos, computer programmes) and group activities, including role-play, helped to hold the participants' interest and encouraged more appropriate gazing behaviours; staring behaviours need to be addressed in people with AS as they are among one of the most frequently observed difficulties (Baron-Cohen *et al.*, 2004; Soyner and Desnoyers Hurley, 1990).

Evaluation of the sociosexual programme (Hénault *et al.*, 2003) revealed that it had helped the participants acquire the technical skills necessary to express emotion (read, decode, and manage emotions), but that they found the actual application of these skills more difficult. This is because individuals with AS tend to get distracted by the details of the face, which makes it more difficult for them to recognize and label an emotion. Recent studies (Channon *et al.*, 2001; Young, 2001) put forward a hypothesis that suggests the presence of amygdalar dysfunction in individuals with AS: the amygdala is the area in the brain responsible for general intelligence and is activated during social recognition exercises. Continued education would be required to help people with AS reduce and organize information related to decoding facial expression, but it is likely that more than this is required to decode emotions.

Several activities were added to the sociosexual programme in order to improve participants' ability to decode facial expressions, and complementary tools were used to improve participants' performance, such as the *Mind-Reading* software (Baron-Cohen *et al.*, 2004), cognitive-behavioural interventions (Attwood, 2003a, 2004a, b), and the Biotouch Interactive Mood Light (Sharper Image Design, 1999). These three tools were specifically aimed at teaching how to read emotions in a face, how to explore and cope with emotions, and how to recognize body signals related to emotional changes, respectively, and they were very helpful for participants.

One limitation of the sociosexual education programme, as with all education and intervention programmes, is the generalizability of gains over the long term; in other words, the ability of the participants to apply the skills they have learned. According to Griffiths *et al.* (1989), generalizability involves support from a therapist, other support networks, and community intervention. First the therapist works on interventions in familiar environments such as home or school. In addition to offering activities in the workshop context, *in vivo* training takes place in everyday settings such as shopping malls or public transport in order to help the individual confront real situations. There is then a second phase when a support network is created (family members, friend, counsellor, youth worker, etc.) that helps to extend one individual's learning, provides them with social support, and maintains the link with the principal therapist. Finally, community interventions such as hobbies, support groups, and other services are offered. Future studies should include these three phases of follow-up to ensure that gains are maintained over the long term.

Support systems also need to be established within existing community services. On several occasions, the researcher's services were requested for therapy and follow-up purposes. The intervention programme therefore opens avenues for creating psychological and sexological services adapted to the specific needs of individuals living with high functioning autism and AS.

In conclusion, researchers and professionals in the fields of specialized education and therapy need to understand the issues involved in the sexuality of individuals with AS. The sexual development and interest in sexuality of people with AS are comparable to those of individuals in the general population. However, their social and sexual profiles differ on several levels: they experience considerable difficulties with social skills, communication, and interpersonal relationships. They present with some needs that could be addressed by sexual education. Intervention programmes specific to their needs must therefore be made available to them.

Evaluation of the programme and results

The programme was evaluated using a variety of measures. The Australian Scale for Asperger's Syndrome (Garnett and Attwood, 1995, as cited in Attwood, 1998a) was used for diagnostic purposes. The Aberrant Behavior Checklist (Aman and Singh, 1986) identified participants' inappropriate behaviours. The Friendship Skills Observation Checklist (Attwood and Gray, 1999a) was used to observe participants' appropriate and inappropriate behaviours in terms of social and personal skills. The sociosexual information questionnaire (Durocher and Fortier, 1999) assessed participants' general knowledge about sexuality before and after they had attended the programme. Finally, the Derogatis Sexual Function Inventory (DSFI) (Derogatis and Melisaratos, 1982) was used to assess, three months after the programme had ended, how participants were applying what they had learned to their daily lives. Because of the intrusive nature of the questionnaire, it was only administered to participants who were over 18 years of age.

It was found that after attending the training programme, the participants' friendship and intimacy skills had significantly increased whereas the frequency of their inappropriate behaviours had decreased (Hénault et al., 2003). Skills such as introducing oneself, making conversation, and engaging in nonverbal communication improved over the course of the programme. Helping and empathetic behaviours were also observed in participants more frequently by the end of the programme. Behaviours of withdrawal and isolation were replaced by a greater reciprocity among group members. The development of friendships among the participants was proof of the growing closeness and openness to others observed during the workshops. Inappropriate behaviours such as inappropriate masturbation, sexual obsessions, voyeurism, fetishism, and exhibitionism decreased. Impulsive behaviours, such as self-mutilation and tantrums, were not significantly represented. At the three month follow-up we found that participants continued to apply their new skills to everyday situations, their general sexual knowledge had increased, and they had a positive attitude towards sexuality.

PART 2

PROGRAMME FOR THE DEVELOPMENT OF SOCIOSEXUAL SKILLS

How to use the programme

The programme is split into 12 workshops tailored to the needs of the participants with AS. The workshops address various topics related to sexuality, and the programme structure is outlined below:

1. Assessment and introduction to the programme.
2. Introduction to sexuality and communication exercises.
3. Love and friendship.
4. Physiological aspects of sexuality.
5. Sexual relations and other sexual behaviours.
6. Emotions.
7. STDs, HIV, and prevention.
8. Sexual orientation.
9. Alcohol, drugs, and sexuality.
10. Sexual abuse and inappropriate sexual behaviours.
11. Sexism and violence in romantic relationships.
12. Managing emotions, theory of mind, and intimacy.

Each workshop begins with an outline of its basic goals and instructions on how it should be structured: topics for discussion, exercises, how the activities work, and how long should be spent on each component. Following this outline, in those workshops that include group discussions, there is an information sheet for the group leader. This provides additional information on the discussion topics and the reactions they may provoke, and ideas on how to guide the discussions (possible questions to pose, etc.).

Many of the activities use worksheets included in the book (including quizzes, information sheets, etc.), which should be photocopied and handed out to participants at the relevant stage of the workshop. These worksheets have a tick in the top right or left corner.

Some workshops include activities that require external resources not provided with this book, for example videos, a website or computer programme, an assessment form or questionnaire from another source, etc. Details of each external resource are given in the references, further reading and resources section at the back of the book. If you plan to use a website (for example Worksheet 11.2., p.176), we recommend that you familiarize yourself with the website before the workshop and ensure that you have downloaded and printed out the relevant sheets and information. Where possible, we have given an alternative activity in case you have difficulty obtaining the resource suggested (e.g. Workshop 6, Activity 1). Where no alternative is given, you may wish to think about a relevant alternative activity yourself.

Almost every workshop will require some preparation on the part of the group leader. For some workshops, this will simply entail ensuring that you have enough photocopies of the activities for every participant. For others, additional preparation will be needed, for example Workshop 6: obtaining photos or images of people expressing different emotions; or Workshop 5: obtaining music, different smells and tastes etc. We therefore strongly recommend that you read through each workshop well in advance to ensure that you are aware of the materials and preparation required.

We recommend that you use appropriate, accurate terminology throughout the programme when referring to genitals, sexual practices, sexual orientation, etc. To avoid any unintentional ambiguity or confusion, we suggest that you use the term "partner" throughout the programme, rather than "boyfriend", "girlfriend", "spouse", etc. It is important to make it clear that the word "couple" can relate to same-sex couples as well as to male–female couples, whether they are married or not.

Finally, during the course of some of the workshops you may be asked (or may wish to inform) about services that exist in your local area, for example sexual health clinics, services for people who have experienced abuse and so on. It is therefore advisable to have up-to-date information on local and national services to hand.

Assessment and introduction to the programme
(**60 minutes**)

The purpose of this first workshop is for the participants to complete the assessment forms and to introduce them to the sociosexual education programme.

Parents and partners of the participants are invited to attend this workshop. During the first part of the session, the group leader provides an introduction to topics covered by the programme and the accompanying materials (exercise sheets, videos, computer software, photographs and images, etc.). The consent form (1.1) and the information sheets (1.2 and 1.3) will then be distributed to, and completed by, the participants. Those under the age of 18 who are not accompanied by a parent take home the consent form for signature and return it in the next workshop. The adult information sheet (1.3) is for those aged 18 years and over. If a participant has not been diagnosed and is not in the process of being diagnosed, but wants to obtain a diagnosis, you may wish to assist him or her in finding a suitable organization or professional to carry out the necessary assessments.

Worksheet 1.4 ("Adolescent questionnaire 1 – Check your knowledge") will also be given to the participants to complete. This worksheet should be completed during the workshop and collected by leaders at the end of the session, ready for group review in Workshop 3.

Worksheet 1.5 "An outline of the course structure" is then distributed to each participant. During the last part of the workshop, questions will be answered and discussion encouraged. Workshop 1 lasts approximately 60 minutes. All subsequent workshops last approximately 90 minutes.

This first workshop allows the participants to become acquainted with the surroundings, establish a first contact with the other group members, and ask questions related to the programme, its duration, and the themes that will be addressed. Worksheets 1.1 to 1.4 comprise all the forms and questionnaires necessary for this first meeting. Adults may be asked to fill in the Derogatis Sexual Function Inventory (DSFI; Derogatis and Meliseratos, 1982), which can be purchased at *www.derogatis-tests.com*. The completed inventory should be returned to the group leader at the end of Workshop 1.

It is advisable for each participant to have a folder in which to file the exercise sheets distributed at each meeting.

✓

1.1 Consent

I agree to participate in the sociosexual skills education skills programme. I understand the different components of the programme. By registering for the programme, I am committing myself to attending all of the workshops.

_____   _____
Participant's signature   Date

_____   _____
Parent's signature (if participants is under 18   Date
years of age)

Confidentiality is assured throughout the project.

Thank you for your cooperation.

✓

1.2 Information sheet – adolescent

1. Name: _____

2. Age: _____

3a. Address: _____

_____

_____

3b. Telephone number: _____

4. Number of years at school: _____

5. Have you received a diagnosis? ☐ Yes ☐ No

    If yes, what is the diagnosis? _____

    When were you diagnosed? _____

    Who gave you the diagnosis? _____

    If no, are you in the process of being diagnosed? _____

6. Do you take medication on a regular basis? ☐ Yes ☐ No

    If yes, which medications do you take and in what dose? _____

    _____

    _____

    _____

N.B. The information you provide will be treated in strict confidence.

Thank you for your cooperation.

✓

1.3 Information sheet – adult

1. Name: _____

2. Age: _____

3a. Address: _____

_____

_____

3b. Telephone number: _____

4a. Occupation: _____

4b. Number of years in education: _____

5. Marital status: ☐ Single ☐ Married ☐ In a relationship ☐ Divorced

6. Have you received a diagnosis? ☐ Yes ☐ No

    If yes, what is the diagnosis? _____

    When were you diagnosed? _____

    Who gave you the diagnosis?_____

    If no, are you in the process of being diagnosed? _____

7. Do you take medication on a regular basis? ☐ Yes ☐ No

If yes, which medications do you take and in what dose? _____

_____

_____

_____

N.B. The information you provide will be treated in strict confidence.

Thank you for your cooperation.

1.4 Adolescent questionnaire 1 – Check your knowledge

Name: _____ Date: _____

Please tick the correct answer for each question.

1. I am the organ that leads to the uterus. I am the passage down which the baby travels at birth. During menstruation, blood flows from me. What am I?
    - (a) penis   ☐
    - (b) vagina   ☐
    - (c) breasts   ☐

2. I am the organ that deposits sperm in a woman's vagina. I get hard during sexual arousal. I am used to urinate and ejaculate. What am I?
    - (a) ovaries   ☐
    - (b) clitoris   ☐
    - (c) penis   ☐

3. We are the glands where sperm is produced. What are we?
    - (a) testicles   ☐
    - (b) vagina   ☐
    - (c) uterus   ☐

4. Do women masturbate?
    - (a) no   ☐
    - (b) yes   ☐

5. A girl can get pregnant during her first sexual encounter, especially if no contraception is used.
    - (a) true   ☐
    - (b) false   ☐

6. Condoms do not protect against STDs (sexually transmitted diseases).
    - (a) true   ☐
    - (b) false   ☐

✔

7.   Homosexuality is a contagious disease.
    (a) true   □
    (b) false   □

8.   Alcohol and drugs improve sexual relations.
    (a) true   □
    (b) false   □

9.   Physical violence is a way of resolving arguments with my girlfriend or boyfriend.
    (a) true   □
    (b) false   □

10. Intimacy is when I talk about my feelings to a person whom I can trust.
    (a) true   □
    (b) false   □

Result: /10

1.5 An outline of the course structure

1. Assessment and introduction to the programme.

2. Introduction to sexuality and communication exercises.

3. Love and friendship.

4. Physiological aspects of sexuality.

5. Sexual relations and other sexual behaviours.

6. Emotions.

7. STDs, HIV, and prevention.

8. Sexual orientation.

9. Alcohol, drugs, and sexuality.

10. Sexual abuse and inappropriate sexual behaviours.

11. Sexism and violence in romantic relationships.

12. Managing emotions, theory of mind, and intimacy.

Introduction to sexuality and communication exercises
(90 minutes)

General goals

To encourage the participants to share their feelings, improve their communication skills, and create a welcoming environment within the group.

1. Presentation of Workshop 2 activities; collect outstanding consent forms (5 minutes).

2. Introduction of individuals in the group: name, age, any other pertinent information (10 minutes).

3. Rules of the workshops: politeness, respect for others, commitment, positive attitude; distribute Worksheet 2.1. Availability of the group leader after each workshop (5 minutes).

4. Warm-up exercise: What is sexuality? (20 minutes). Spend five minutes brainstorming in small teams (words, phrases, images that come up in response to the question "What is sexuality"). Teams then share their ideas with the others in the group. At the end, ask the participants how they found the exercise and where they learned these words and phrases (newspapers, radio, television, books, classes, etc.). Congratulate each team and introduce the second exercise.

5. Communication exercise (inspired by Kempton 1993) (20 minutes). Divide the group into two smaller groups. The participants in the first group place themselves in a circle (back to back) and the others form a circle around them, facing them. Those in the outer circle must ask the following questions to those in the inner circle. Those in the inner circle should talk about each of the questions for a period of one minute:
    - What scares you in life?
    - What makes you the most happy?
    - With whom do you enjoy spending time?

After each question, the individuals on the outside circle must rotate to the right. Then swap the groups around.

Conclusion

Remind participants of the goals of the meeting and congratulate the efforts of each participant. Answer any questions.

2.1 Behaviours and skills encouraged during group discussions

1. Demonstrating interest towards other participants through eye contact and listening.

2. Waiting for others to have finished their thoughts before speaking.

3. Giving your own opinion and defending your own point of view.

4. Providing constructive criticism and suggestions.

5. Learning to decode the intentions of others.

Love and friendship
(90 minutes)

General goals

To have the participants identify and recognize characteristics related to love and friendship and those that they would like to find in a partner.

1. Review "Adolescent Questionnaire 1 – Check your knowledge" (Worksheet 1.4) (15 minutes).

2a. Discussion: what are the differences between love and friendship? Psychological and emotional.

2b. Discussion: what are you attracted to in another person (physical, psychological, and emotional characteristics; personality; affinities, etc.)? See the discussion questions proposed in 3.1, "Information for the group leader" (20 minutes).

3. Activity: "My values in interpersonal relationships" (Worksheet 3.2) (15 minutes).

4. Activity: "The personal columns game" (Worksheet 3.3). Analyse two ads: "Kiki" and "Young 25-year-old guy". Do you think these people are seeking love or friendship? How do we decode these types of ads? (15 minutes)

5. Activity: "Wanted" (Worksheet 3.4). Create your own personal ad, describing yourself (qualities, strengths, characteristics) and what you would like in a friend or partner (20 minutes). The goal of this activity is to "break the ice" in order to know yourself better and identify the characteristics desired in someone you like.

 Source material: Durocher, L. and Fortier, M. (1999) *Programme d'éducation sexuelle des Centres jeunesse de Montréal.* Montréal: Le Centre jeunesse de Montréal – Institut Universitaire.

3.1 Information for the group leader

The goal of this workshop is to foster growth in participants' interpersonal relationships and sexuality by giving them the opportunity to explore the different facets of adolescent sexuality. By providing them with the skills and knowledge necessary for healthy human relationships, they will be in a better position to protect themselves and others. Aims include the following:

1. Developing participants' capacity to think and talk about various aspects of sexuality. Identifying values with respect to love, friendship, and sexuality, and reflecting on and sharing these values.

2. Leading the participants to believe that their personal opinion is as important as that of their partner. Providing them with skills, such as practical tips and tools to facilitate discussion or initiate activities that will enable them to communicate more effectively with their partner.

3. Leading the participants to respect the differences and opinions of others. Introducing them to various healthy and positive behaviours related to sexuality.

Discussion questions

- What are the characteristics of a potential or ideal partner?

- What do you find attractive in another person?

- What is needed to fall in love? To be attracted to another person? To feel excited?

- Is it difficult to describe oneself, name one's own qualities, etc.?

- What are your strengths, the things at which you excel? How would you describe yourself?

Source material: Durocher, L. and Fortier, M. (1999) *Programme d'éducation sexuelle des Centres jeunesse de Montréal.* 121
Montréal: Le Centre jeunesse de Montréal – Institut Universitaire.

✓

3.2 My values in interpersonal relationships

By establishing what is important in your life you can become aware that values, according to how you rate their importance and how you use them in interpersonal relationships, vary from one person to the next. Rate the values below by writing the numbers 1 (most important to you) to 18 (least important to you) in the boxes. Do this exercise on your own and then compare your responses with those of the other participants. This will perhaps enable you to understand one another better.

☐	Self-respect	☐	Honesty
☐	Respect of others	☐	Fidelity
☐	Beauty	☐	Sharing
☐	Fun	☐	Intelligence
☐	Friendship	☐	Sexuality
☐	Freedom	☐	Self-confidence
☐	Love	☐	Sense of humour
☐	Curiosity	☐	Tenderness
☐	Happiness	☐	Equality

3.3 The personal columns game

Hi. My name is Kiki. I'm 25 years old with brown hair and eyes. I'm real cool and laid back. I'm looking for a guy that's laid back like me, who likes music, going out, hiking in the woods, and a little bit of everything. By the way, I'm looking for a musician too, if you're interested. If you want to reach me, my voice mail number is 3058.

Young guy, 25 years old, likes rock music, ATV, motorbikes, restaurants, movies, nature, looking for young guy 18–20 years old, cool, who knows what he wants, for stable relationship, long-term, sincere, not complicated. Phone 4219.

✓

3.4 "Wanted"

Goal

To identify and describe the characteristics that you would like to find in a friend or partner.

Hi, my name is…

I'm looking for a person who…

Physiological aspects of sexuality
(90 minutes)

General goals

To review basic notions of anatomy, particularly of male and female genitalia (function, characteristics, structure). To lead participants to talk about the anatomical, physiological, and psychological aspects of sexuality while fostering a positive self-image.

1.   Review of previous workshop; discussion and participants' experience (10 minutes).

"What does it mean to be an adult?"

2.   Discussion of sexual maturity, functions of the genitals and reproduction (desire for children, physical sensations related to sexuality, phases of the sexual response cycle, etc.) (30 minutes). See 4.1, "Information for the group leader".

3.   Present the figure of the sexual response cycle and discuss the phases of sexual response (20 minutes) (Worksheet 4.2).

4.   Activity: labelling diagrams of male and female genitals. Either by writing directly on the sheets or by using the labels on Worksheet 4.3, participants label the diagrams of genitals on Worksheets 4.4 and 4.6. This will demonstrate how much biological knowledge they already have (Worksheets 4.5 and 4.7 show the correctly labelled diagrams.). Discuss the functions of each of the organs (Worksheet 4.8) (30 minutes).

Source material: Durocher, L. and Fortier, M. (1999) *Programme d'éducation sexuelle des Centres jeunesse de Montréal.* 125
Montréal: Le Centre jeunesse de Montréal – Institut Universitaire.

4.1 Information for the group leader

By facilitating discussions about changes in adolescents, this workshop introduces different themes within sexual education. The transition from puberty to adulthood raises several questions for participants. Understanding the anatomical, physiological, and psychological changes related to puberty can help adolescents cope with concerns and react positively to the changes taking place within them. The materials and activities presented in this workshop were created to address these concerns by encouraging participants to express their feelings and worries and to play an active role in searching for answers to their questions.

It is difficult for teenage participants to deal with very personal topics in an open and intimate manner, and they may find discussing them very intimidating. Some adolescents become silent and claim to know everything about anatomy when it is time to talk about their changing bodies. It is therefore up to the group leader to establish a dialogue on questions related to puberty. Here are some suggestions which might be used to facilitate discussion.

- Use language that is precise and easy to understand.

- Define new terms and provide practical information and examples.

- Create an atmosphere that will allow the participants to feel comfortable asking questions and talking about their experiences and their feelings.

- Encourage them to express themselves in their own words. Accept popular language but favour the use of appropriate terminology.

- Be receptive to all kinds of emotions.

- Consider their opinions and recognize that they have some knowledge. However, don't assume that they know everything because they are 14, 15, or 16 years old or older. Start with what they know and enhance their knowledge.

If you adopt this approach, teenage participants will understand what is happening, will be reassured, and will not feel alone with their questions, concerns, and experiences. They need to have confirmation that it is OK to develop at their own pace – they are full of questions and new feelings and often wonder if they are normal.

In addition to being given objective information about their bodies, adolescents need to feel free to talk about their values, feelings, and concerns related to their gender.

In summary, this workshop invites each participant to feel more comfortable with the reality of being an adolescent. The following activities will trigger discussions about puberty; this can lead some participants to share personal experiences, while others will find the answers to some of their questions.

126   Source material: Durocher, L. and Fortier, M. (1999) *Programme d'éducation sexuelle des Centres jeunesse de Montréal.* Montréal: Le Centre jeunesse de Montréal – Institut Universitaire.

Goals of this workshop

The goals of this workshop are to discuss the anatomical, physiological, and psychological experiences that adolescents have concerning their sexuality while fostering a positive self-image among participants.

- Lead the young people to describe the anatomical, physiological, and psychological changes that accompany puberty.

- Identify the internal organs and external genitals of males and females and understand their functions.

- Help participants to understand the physical changes that take place during puberty.

- Describe the body's new capacities acquired during puberty.

- Help participants to understand the different aspects of sexual awakening.

- Encourage participants to acquire a positive attitude and self-image about the changes that take place during puberty.

- Present the ways in which adolescents' sexual growth and change are manifested.

- Lead the participants to realize that psychological and physical changes do not occur at the same time and in the same way for everyone.

- Situate puberty in the context of a lifetime of physical and psychological change.

- Discuss the fears and joys associated with the physical and psychological changes that take place during puberty.

Questions for discussion

1. What are the differences between a child and an adolescent? What are the differences between an adolescent and an adult?

2. Brainstorming activity: invite the participants to generate words that they use to discuss or refer to the genitals of men and women, or those used with respect to any other activity related to sexuality. Then ask them to find the factual term related to each of the words (e.g. "masturbation", "vulva", "penis", "intercourse", etc.).

3. Finish the activity by emphasizing that using the factual term to designate the various genitals or reproductive organs, or any other subject related to sexuality, is a sign of respect that also facilitates communication and comprehension.

Source material: Durocher, L. and Fortier, M. (1999) *Programme d'éducation sexuelle des Centres jeunesse de Montréal.* 127
Montréal: Le Centre jeunesse de Montréal – Institut Universitaire.

4.2 Sexual response cycle

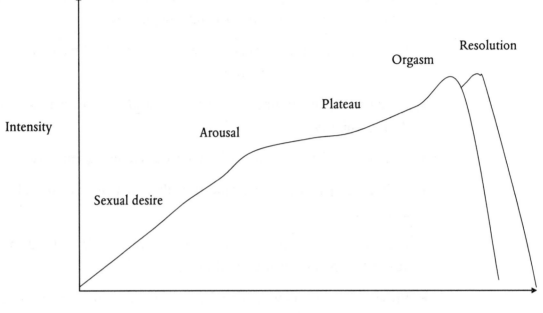

Adapted from Masters and Johnson (1968)

Phases of sexual response

1. Sexual desire: feelings of being drawn to another.

2. Arousal: male – erection; female – vaginal lubrication.

3. Plateau: arousal stabilizes and then increases; sexual tension increases.

4. Orgasm: involuntary contractions of the pelvic muscles, lasts 5–15 seconds.

5. Resolution: decrease in arousal and return to the resting phase (refractory period).

Male: During the refractory period he is unable to respond to new sexual stimulation.

Female: During the refractory period there is a possibility that she can be aroused again and have more than one orgasm.

4.3 List of urogenital organs of the male and female

scrotum	uterus
testicles	anus
penis	cervix
clitoris	glans
vas deferens	anus
penis	urinary meatus
vaginal opening	glans
labia minora	vagina
sperm	fallopian tubes
labia majora	ovary
prostate	vulva
urethra	scrotum
ovum	urinary meatus

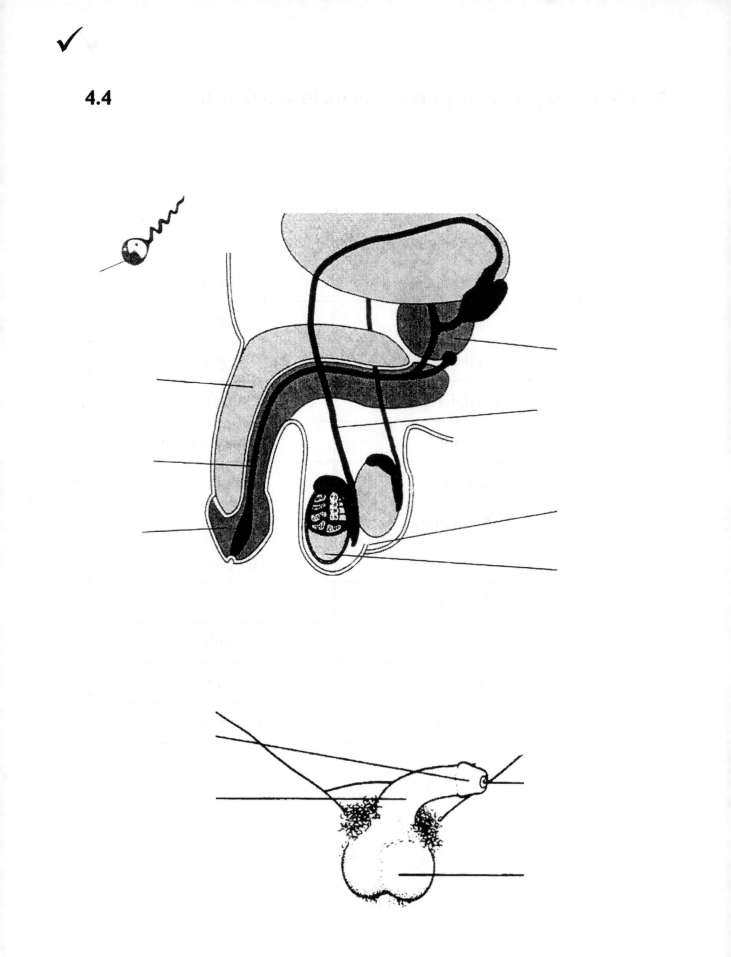

4.5

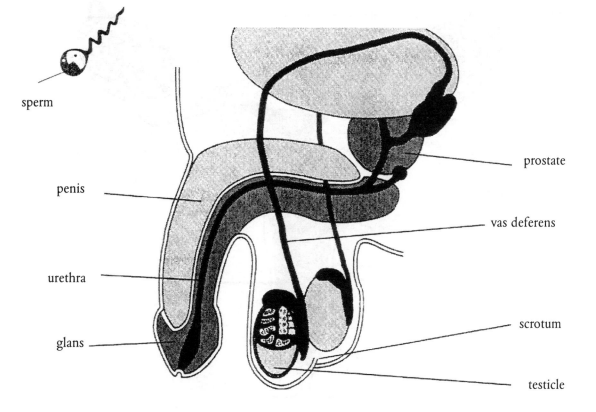

sperm

penis

urethra

glans

prostate

vas deferens

scrotum

testicle

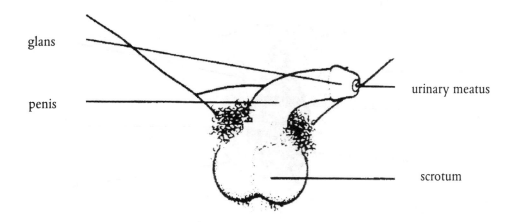

glans

penis

urinary meatus

scrotum

4.6

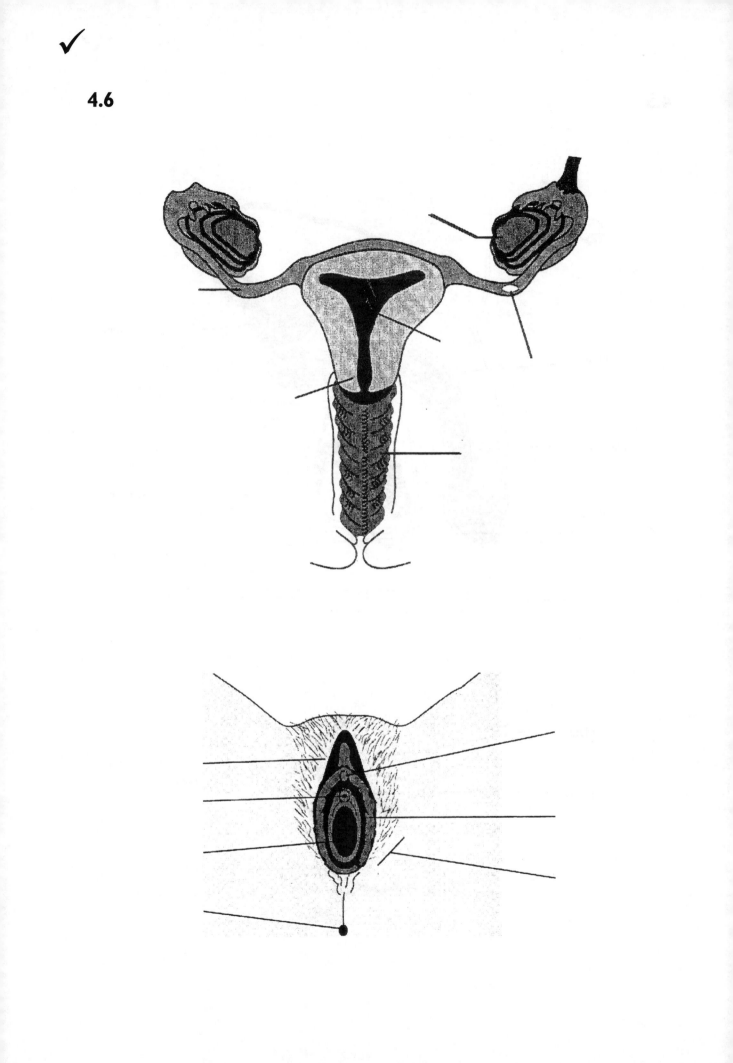

4.7

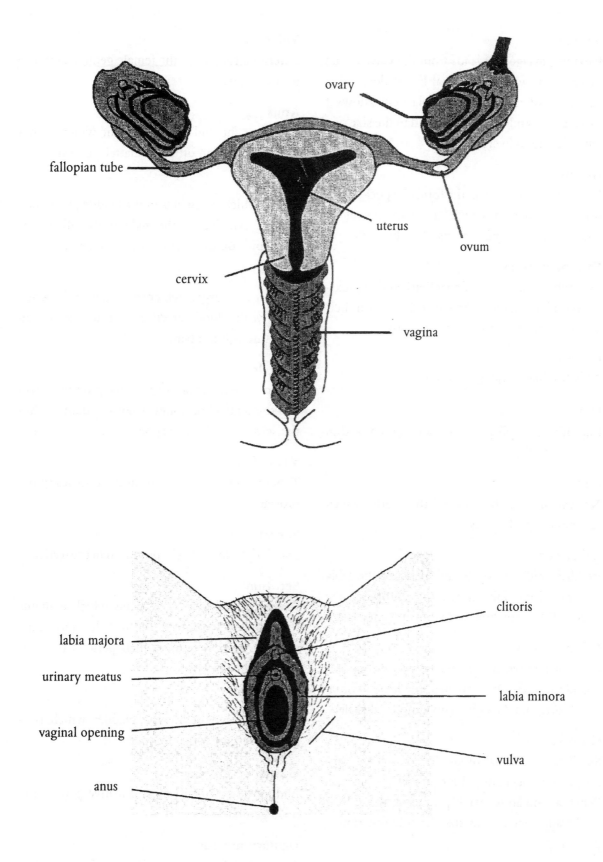

ovary

fallopian tube

uterus

ovum

cervix

vagina

clitoris

labia majora

urinary meatus

labia minora

vaginal opening

vulva

anus

4.8 Functions of the urogenital organs

Vagina

Flexible passage that leads from the vulva to the uterus from which menstrual blood flows. The vagina is not very wide but its elasticity allows it to adapt to penile penetration and to the size of a baby during delivery.

Uterus

Internal female organ in the form of a pocket. It is the organ within which the baby develops during the first nine months of its life.

Fallopian tubes

Two tubes, the width of spaghetti, and approximately 10 cm long, which lead the ova on their passage from the ovaries to the uterus.

Ovaries

Glands which produce the ova.

Ovum

Reproductive cell produced and stored within the ovaries. (Plural: "ova".)

Cervix

Narrow area at the base of the uterus which secretes cervical mucus.

Labia minora

Reddish folds of skin found inside of the labia majora which join above the clitoris. They appear differently from one woman to the next.

Labia majora

Folds of skin which are covered by hair on their outside surface. Once opened, the labia minora, the clitoris, and the vaginal opening are revealed.

Clitoris

Small female sexual organ. The clitoris is very sensitive to touch. At puberty, it increases in size. When a woman is sexually aroused, the clitoris swells and increases in size. Its sole function is pleasure.

Vulva

Exterior structure of the female genital, entrance to the vagina.

Anus

Orifice at the end of the intestine which allows for the expulsion of faecal matter (faeces).

Urethra

Canal, which originates in the bladder, by which urine is expelled. In the male, it also allows for the expulsion of semen during ejaculation.

Penis

Male sexual organ which becomes rigid when filled with blood (erection). Urine and semen flow through the penis.

Testicles

Two oval shaped male organs that produce sperm and the sexual hormones. They are found within the scrotum and are very sensitive.

Vas deferens

Tubes which lead sperm from the testicles to the prostate.

Sperm

Small reproductive cells produced in the testicles.

Scrotum

Pouch located below the penis which contains the testicles. It protects the testicles and keeps them at a temperature which permits them to produce healthy sperm.

Prostate

Gland situated below the bladder which produces a large part of the sperm.

Glans

Ending of the penis; most sensitive part of the male genital.

Urinary meatus

Extremity of the urinary canal where urine is expelled and sperm is ejected.

Sexual relations and other sexual behaviours
(90 minutes)

General goals

To lead each participant to describe what a sexual relation is to him/her, name different kinds of sexual behaviour, and identify reasons for having sexual relations.

1. Fears: the goal is to allow the participants to express the fears that they may have about sexual relations (see 5.1, "Information for the group leader"). Participants should fill in Worksheet 5.2 and have a group discussion (25 minutes).

2. A sexual encounter: the goal of the next exercise is to think about what could make a sexual encounter agreeable and pleasant. Participants should fill in Worksheet 5.3 and have a group discussion (25 minutes).

3. The five senses: hyposensitivity, hypersensitivity, acceptable or normal sensitivity – what impact can these have on sexuality? What are the possible means by which this impact can be decreased? Test the participants' different senses using the methods explained under "The five senses related to sexuality" (p.137) and listed on Worksheet 5.4. Discuss tips to help deal with participants' sensitivities (40 minutes).

Source material: Durocher, L. and Fortier, M. (1999) *Programme d'éducation sexuelle des Centres jeunesse de Montréal.* 135
Montréal: Le Centre jeunesse de Montréal – Institut Universitaire.

5.1 Information for the group leader

This worksheet provides the group leader with the necessary information to help lead this topic. However, it should be noted that the group leader is by far the most important factor in enabling the goals of this topic to be met. Inevitably, as group leader, you will be asked personal questions. It is important to be prepared for these and to refuse all questions that you judge to be too personal.

You, like the participants, may at times feel uncomfortable talking about sexual relations, since this is indeed an intimidating topic. We suggest that you share your discomfort with the young people, which will help to decrease any tension. A touch of humour will often help too… we also ask that the group leader respect the choice of certain adolescents who might prefer to remain silent.

Nonetheless, you should establish a candid dialogue on sexuality and avoid making value judgements. It is likely that questions will be asked to which you will not know the answer. You can take advantage of such a situation by inviting participants to find out extra information and remind them that learning about sexuality is a lifelong process.

Important factors must be considered throughout these activities, such as the age of the adolescents, their maturity and sexual history. In addition, cultural and ethnic factors should be addressed. It should be noted that cultural differences exist with respect to premarital sex, and these should be considered when discussing such topics as virginity or rupture of the hymen (an intact hymen can be viewed as a symbol of virginity). Circumcision is also frequently performed a few days after birth within certain religious contexts.

The information provided and the vocabulary and means used to convey it must be adjusted according to the characteristics of the group. You should note that some adolescents in the group may not be sexually active while others may be. The interests, concerns, and questions raised may therefore be quite different within the same group. Regardless of whether they are sexually active or not, discussing this topic will allow the participants to become better prepared to experience their first or next sexual relation.

Throughout the activities, the group leader must be sensitive to fact that adolescents commonly have several fears about romantic and sexual relationships. The topic may induce feelings of guilt in some adolescents. To prepare yourself to discuss this topic, consider these common questions and fears that preoccupy young people:

- Will he find me attractive?
- Who makes the first moves?
- Is my penis big enough?
- How do I know if the other person likes it?
- Will it hurt me?

 Source material: Durocher, L. and Fortier, M. (1999) *Programme d'éducation sexuelle des Centres jeunesse de Montréal.* Montréal: Le Centre jeunesse de Montréal – Institut Universitaire.

- Will I be disappointed?
- Can you tell if it's someone's first time?
- Will everyone notice?
- Will I ejaculate too quickly?
- Will I be able to get a "hard-on"?
- Will I have an orgasm?
- Do I have enough/too much hair?
- How am I going to suggest using a condom? Will he accept?
- I'm afraid of getting pregnant...
- I'm afraid that I won't live up to it...
- I'm afraid of catching some disease...
- I'm afraid that he/she will leave me afterwards...
- I'm afraid to disappoint...
- Will my parents notice?
- How will I go about it?
- Will he/she tell his/her friends all about it?

All of these concerns are frequently encountered. Adolescents need to be reassured and to have some of their fears reduced to realistic proportions. It is helpful for them to know that the level of satisfaction in first sexual relations is rarely high. Sexuality is learned by trial and error and is tied into a process of discovering one's self and partner.

The five senses related to sexuality

The information outlined in this section is background to Worksheet 5.4.

To the author's knowledge no studies to date have examined the link between sensory states and sexuality in AS. Given the intimate link between sexuality and the senses, this omission is certainly puzzling, especially in light of the fact that individuals with AS can experience hyper- or hyposensitivity.

Hypersensitivity can be defined as extreme sensitivity experienced in one or more of the five senses. Auditory and tactile hypersensitivity are common in AS and may be associated with neurological disorders. For example, light background music played at a low volume can be perceived as loud and shrill. Similarly, a slight brushing up against the skin can provoke the same intensity of pain as would be caused by a sharp object. Various forms of sexual stimulation can therefore cause discomfort or even pain for individuals with AS, reinforcing avoidance behaviours and hindering the development of intimate relationships.

Source material: Durocher, L. and Fortier, M. (1999) *Programme d'éducation sexuelle des Centres jeunesse de Montréal.* 137
Montréal: Le Centre jeunesse de Montréal – Institut Universitaire.

In contrast, hyposensitivity can be defined as weak sensory responses to modest forms of stimulation. In this case, multiple exposures to stimuli are necessary to experience the sensation as a whole.

The five senses activity described in Worksheet 5.4 was devised in order to explore sensory responses to various experiences so that individuals with AS will be better equipped to identify and avoid stimulations that could lead to sensory confusion. The goal of the exercise is to test each of the five senses and tick the appropriate box to determine the level of sensitivity experienced. For example, what is the individual's reaction to soft music or to a loud noise? This can be tested by placing headphones over his or her ears and playing soft and loud music through them (i.e. classical music and hard rock), or whispering in his/her ear and slamming a door. The sensory reaction is usually quite marked. In order to test the sense of touch, the forearm can be caressed with a plush fabric or fur. The exercise should then be repeated using sandpaper. Examples are provided for each sense that needs to be tested. This experiment will allow the participant to express what he or she feels and to realize that what is perceived by his or her senses has an impact on behaviour. The second part of the activity examines the impact of sensory responses on sexuality. These questions can be useful starting points in addressing the subject of sexual behaviours.

Goals of this workshop

The goal of this workshop is for the participants to know and understand some of the different aspects related to sexual relations.

- Allow participants to describe what the term "sexual relations" means to them, and how important sexual relations are for them.

- Have them talk about the different forms that sexual relations can take.

- Allow them to identify factors which motivate individuals to engage in sexual relations.

- Enrich their understanding of various aspects of sexual relations, e.g. emotional aspects, physical aspects, etc.

- Allow them to identify the different types of pleasure related to sexual relations.

- Identify myths about sexual relations.

- Have them identify and name the conditions that are necessary for an enriching sexual experience.

138   Source material: Durocher, L. and Fortier, M. (1999) *Programme d'éducation sexuelle des Centres jeunesse de Montréal.* Montréal: Le Centre jeunesse de Montréal – Institut Universitaire.

5.2 Fears

Here is a list of common fears about romantic relationships and sexual relations. Circle the letter corresponding to any fears that you have had.

A	Fear of not being liked	**M**	Fear of regretting it
B	Fear of being compared	**N**	Fear that it will hurt
C	Fear of being disappointed	**O**	Fear of getting naked in front of someone
D	Fear of not knowing what to say or do	**P**	Fear of catching a disease
E	Fear of being turned down	**Q**	Fear of pregnancy
F	Fear of showing my lack of experience	**R**	Fear of not getting a "hard-on"
G	Fear of disappointing	**S**	Fear of ejaculating too quickly
H	Fear of looking "easy"	**T**	Fear that my body is not nice enough (legs, stomach, penis, breasts, hair, muscles)
I	Fear of it being too intimate	**U**	Fear of not having an orgasm
J	Fear of what others will think	**V**	Fear of being left afterwards
K	Fear of being provocative	**W**	Fear that the other person will tell everything
L	Fear that the other person only wants sex	**X Y Z**	Other fears (give examples)

If you circled ten or more fears, you're in the norm. Don't stay alone with your fears. Talk about them: they'll be less scary.

✓

5.3 A sexual encounter…

…is fun…

WHEN we are ready; that is, when the need and desire for it really comes from us and not from external pressures.

WHEN what we do is in agreement with our value system.

WHEN we choose someone who we like and whom we desire, love, or care about.

WHEN we feel good with our partner and can fulfil our needs for tenderness, fun, and communication.

WHEN we take time to get to know one another, talk about what we like, our feelings.

WHEN we know and like our body as well as the other person's body.

WHEN we take our time.

WHEN we are attuned to our needs and those of the other person.

WHEN we explore our capacity to "let go" in an encounter without desperately seeking an orgasm.

WHEN we use a good method of contraception (if we don't want a baby).

WHEN we protect ourselves from STDs.

…is less fun…

WHEN we have no feelings for the other person, don't respect them, or don't worry about them.

WHEN we have sexual relations more often than we really want and get very little pleasure out of them.

WHEN we have sexual relations because of peer pressure or to prove that we are no different than anyone else.

WHEN we always do it quickly for fear of getting caught.

WHEN we do it only to make the other person happy.

WHEN we go against our principles.

WHEN we don't use birth control and don't want a baby.

WHEN we don't talk before, during, or after, and we don't give ourselves the chance to be more sexually fulfilled.

WHEN we don't protect ourselves from STDs.

What makes a sexual encounter fun for you?

5.4 The five senses

	Hyposensitive Under-sensitive	Sensitive Acceptable	Hypersensitive Over-sensitive
1. Hearing (soft music/loud noise)			
2. Smell (perfume/alcohol)			
3. Touch (soft fabric/sandpaper)			
4. Sight (bright colours/blurry images)			
5. Taste (lemon/honey or chocolate)			

What impact does your level of sensitivity have on your sexuality?

_____

_____

_____

_____

Can you think of possible ways and means of tackling under-/over- sensitivity?

_____

_____

_____

_____

Emotions
(90 minutes)

General goals

To help participants to be able to recognize different emotions and use this skill in daily life; to help participants identify the intensity of emotions and assist them in thinking about and acting on others' mental states and attitudes.

The whole group participates in the first activity. Then separate the group into two teams of five or six individuals to complete Activities 2 and 3 respectively.

1. Present the photos in the *SexoTrousse* (Lemay, 1996): Each participant must name the emotion on each human face and describe a context in which they might feel that emotion. Next, mime the of one the emotions and ask the other group participants to guess what it is; then it's the participants' turn to mime emotions and have the group guess what they are (20 minutes).

   Instead, you can also take pictures of the faces of men and women expressing basic emotions – joy, anger, sadness, fear, neutral, surprise, anxiety – and present them as specified above. It is preferable to use photographs, since they are more realistic, rather than drawings or pictograms. Photographs from the Emotions Library in the *Mind-Reading* software (Baron-Cohen *et al.*, 2004) could be used for this workshop.

2. Role-play: One after the other, each participant picks an emotion card (Worksheet 6.1) and mimes its content without using language (i.e. using nonverbal skills). Meanwhile, the other group participants must guess which emotions are being mimed (45 minutes).

3. *Gaining Face* software (Team Asperger, 2000): Use the five activities presented in the CD-Rom (including the final quiz) to measure each participant's performance. Note the results obtained by each participant. The *Mind-Reading* software (Baron-Cohen *et al.*, 2004) can also be used for this activity (45 minutes).

4. Optional activity: Ask each participant to look at Worksheet 6.2 at regular intervals throughout the course and beyond and answer the thought-provoking questions 2 and 3. The Biotouch Interactive Mood Light (Sharper Image Design, 1999) can also be used. Follow the instructions in Chapter 3, p.71.

6.1 Emotion cards

I have a headache – I'm grumpy	It's boring today because it's raining
Oh! What a beautiful birthday cake!	I was startled when I saw you
My heart is beating very fast because I have to meet with my boss	I'm worried because my friend is sick
My friend hurt my feelings	I feel good when my friend is there
My mind is at ease, I got good medical results	I'm disappointed because my friend didn't come to the restaurant
I'm worried. I don't have enough money to pay the rent	I have fun when I participate in an evening
My heart pounds when we go too fast in the car	I tremble when I walk alone on the street at night
I feel comfortable because it's going well at work	I'm happy with myself because I did a good job
I'm happy because my friend gave me a gift	I run away when people in my class argue
I don't like people making jokes about me – I get angry easily	I'm bad and aggressive because my teacher doesn't agree with me

✓

6.2 Thinking about emotions

Exercises

Hello! Here are some questions for you to answer. There are no right or wrong answers. What *you* write is important. You don't have to use all of the lines, just write what you have to say. Have fun and use your imagination!

QUESTION 1

How do you feel during the sexual education workshops?

_____

_____

_____

_____

_____

_____

QUESTION 2

Tick the emotions or feelings that you are feeling right now. You can tick more than one emotion.

Happy   ☐

Cheerful   ☐

Neutral   ☐

Sad   ☐

Angry   ☐

Irritated   ☐

Distracted   ☐

Tired   ☐

Other _____

QUESTION 3

Describe why you are feeling these emotions. There may be more then one reason why you feel this way.

_____

_____

_____

_____

_____

_____

_____

_____

_____

_____

_____

_____

_____

_____

_____

_____

_____

_____

_____

_____

_____

_____

_____

_____

_____

STDs, HIV, and prevention
(90 minutes)

General goals

To provide participants with the necessary knowledge and skills to prevent sexually transmitted disease and unwanted pregnancy. To develop a sense of responsibility within their sexuality and to encourage effective and appropriate contraceptive use adapted to their lifestyles.

1. Introduction to the topic and presentation of specific implications of unprotected sexual relations. Ask the participants why they think protection is important. Ask them to name the STDs that they know about, their symptoms, and the different contraceptives available (15 minutes) (see 7.1, "Information for the group leader").

2. "Quiz on contraception and prevention" (15 minutes) (Worksheet 7.2). Participants should complete the sheet and then discuss the answers.

3. "Without a condom, it's no" (15 minutes) (Worksheet 7.3). The group should discuss the answers after participants have completed the sheet.

4. Demonstration on model of penis: "How to use a condom: step by step" (25 minutes) (Worksheet 7.4). The group leader or a participant should review the seven steps in consecutive order.

5. Use Worksheet 7.5, "Risk of transmission of HIV and STDs" as a means of generating discussion (20 minutes). This activity can be replaced by a film/documentary on the prevention of STDs or the video *Under Cover Dick* from Diverse City Press at *www.diverse-city.com* (Hingsburger 1996).

 Source material: Durocher, L. and Fortier, M. (1999) *Programme d'éducation sexuelle des Centres jeunesse de Montréal.* Montréal: Le Centre jeunesse de Montréal – Institut Universitaire.

7.1 Information for the group leader

From the start, you, as group leader, must broach this topic and get each participant engaged in talking about contraception and the prevention of STDs and HIV. The first activity is therefore very important. The activities have been developed to involve boys and girls and men and women equally, since this guide encourages joint responsibility for contraception.

As group leader you must, at all times, take care to present sexuality within a positive light. It is of utmost importance that the discourse on this topic be positive, open, and non-judgemental. Respect for different ideas must be apparent in your conversation and nonverbal communication in order to stimulate openness in participants' discussions and exchanges. The personal lives of the adolescents must, at all times, be protected. They should know, from the beginning, that they do not have to divulge any personal experiences.

Despite the numerous prevention programmes available, some adolescents and adults will fail to use contraception during their sexual encounters. Sexual education programmes should empower participants to make responsible choices about contraception, and provide the necessary information and tools to help them prevent unwanted pregnancy and STDs. It is important to recognize that adolescents may already have (mis)information and reservations regarding contraception and the prevention of STDs and HIV. It is therefore crucial to correct any myths and false beliefs that they may hold. In addition to sharing accurate information with them, you must encourage them to participate actively in, and persevere with, negotiations of safe sex and birth control while acknowledging the challenges that this poses to their budding sexual lives.

The goal is not for participants to remember every detail about each method of contraception, but for them to retain the information that will allow them to make wise choices, use contraceptives in a correct manner, debunk myths related to prevention (of STDs and pregnancy), and encourage them to make use of health services in their search for contraception.

It is important that the activities take place in a fun and pleasant atmosphere. Therefore, when it is time to demonstrate the different contraceptives, it is important to allow participants to express their embarrassment through laughter and jokes. This will subsequently facilitate a more serious discussion.

Source material: Durocher, L. and Fortier, M. (1999) *Programme d'éducation sexuelle des Centres jeunesse de Montréal.* 147
Montréal: Le Centre jeunesse de Montréal – Institut Universitaire.

Goals of this workshop

To provide participants with the knowledge necessary for them to use contraceptives effectively and appropriately.

- Add to participants' existing knowledge of contraception and the prevention of STDs, HIV and unwanted pregnancy.

- Encourage them to express their feelings about the various methods of contraception.

- Discuss male and female responsibility regarding contraception.

- Participants should know where information and services related to contraception and the prevention of STDs, HIV and unwanted pregnancy are available, free, and confidential.

- They should learn to value condom use both as a method of contraception and in the prevention of STDs and HIV.

- Alert them to the importance of protecting themselves and others.

148   Source material: Durocher, L. and Fortier, M. (1999) *Programme d'éducation sexuelle des Centres jeunesse de Montréal.* Montréal: Le Centre jeunesse de Montréal – Institut Universitaire.

7.2 Quiz on contraception and prevention

Young people may have unplanned or irregular sex and may not use contraceptives to prevent sexually transmitted diseases (STDs) and unwanted pregnancy. The information you have about this topic is very important because it allows you to make appropriate choices in your sexual life. Pick up your pencil and complete this quiz! Maybe you'll learn something new. Ask your course leader if you are unsure about any of the points in the quiz.

1. "Natural" methods, such as the "calendar method", are not recommended for adolescents.
   - ☐ true
   - ☐ false

2. There is a risk of pregnancy when ejaculation occurs near the vulva.
   - ☐ true
   - ☐ false

3. Condoms are an effective method of contraception for preventing STDs.
   - ☐ true
   - ☐ false

4. The morning-after pill can be taken up to three days after unprotected sexual relations.
   - ☐ true
   - ☐ false

5. The pre-ejaculate contains a sufficient amount of sperm for there to be a possibility of fertilization.
   - ☐ true
   - ☐ false

6. The contraceptive pill is very effective at preventing pregnancy when taken correctly.
   - ☐ true
   - ☐ false

7. The contraceptive pill does not protect against STDs.
   - ☐ true
   - ☐ false

8. Condoms cannot be re-used.
   - ☐ true
   - ☐ false

9. Adolescents are fertile from the beginning of puberty (girls: first period; boys: beginning of sperm production).
   - ☐ true
   - ☐ false

10. The morning-after pill and abortions are emergency measures and not methods of contraception.
    - ☐ true
    - ☐ false

You can't always tell if someone is using contraception.
Make sure you know about methods of contraception
and when and how to use them!

✓

7.3 "Without a condom, it's no"

Tick the excuses that you think are the most commonly used when someone is trying to avoid using a condom…

- ☐ "There's no risk of AIDS or STDs: those are just stories…"
- ☐ "Don't be afraid: it's not dangerous at our age…"
- ☐ "If you really love me, you'll want to…"
- ☐ "If you don't want to, it's over between us…"
- ☐ "You're not cool! Just once without a condom…"
- ☐ "We're faithful to one another, we don't need a condom…"
- ☐ "It's not real sex if there's no penetration…"
- ☐ "Trust me! I don't need a condom…"
- ☐ "Nobody in the gang uses condoms…"

Have you come across any other excuses?

What could you answer to remain responsible and proud of yourself in the face of this pressure?

7.4 How to use a condom: step by step

1. **Check the expiry date printed on the package or box. Carefully open the package so as not to damage the condom**. Be careful of rings, nails, teeth, etc. which may tear or damage the condom. Condoms can be bought at the pharmacy, corner store, in vending machines, or in a sex shop (in the case of novelty condoms). There are several brands, of which the main ones are: Ramses, Durex, Sheik, Shields, Nuform, Prime, Beyond, Trojan. Condoms may have different characteristics: they may be ribbed, textured, or super thin. Some condoms contain a spermicide. All these varieties enable couples to pick the condom which best suits their needs. For better protection against STDs use lubricated latex condoms. They are more resistant and do not let through the majority of bacteria and viruses that cause STDs, such as HIV. This is not the case for natural membrane condoms such as Fourex, Naturalamb and 4X Trojan.

    Condoms are sold as a single unit or in packs of 3, 12, 24, and 36. Always check the expiry date that is shown on the package. Discoloured or sticky latex condoms, or condoms that came from damaged boxes or yellowed packets, should not be used.

2. **Check the unrolling direction**. The ring must be on the outside.

3. **Place the condom on the glans of the erect penis before any contact with the partner's genitals occurs**.

4. **Pinch the tip of the condom to remove the air**. The majority of condoms on the market have a reservoir tip, but if there isn't one, leave a space to collect the semen.

5. **Unroll the condom to the base of the penis**.

6. **Use a water-based lubricant**. Vaseline, baby oil, or Crisco oil should never be used as they may damage latex. The use of a lubricant decreases friction and the risk that the condom will break, and it may increase sensitivity. A spermicide, such as nonoxynol-9, may also be used to increase protection against HIV and STDs. Spermicides can also serve as a lubricant. Avoid a nonoxynol-9-based spermicide for anal sex because it irritates the anal mucosa.

7. **After ejaculation, remove the penis, while holding the condom at the base, to avoid any leakage of semen which could occur with loss of erection**.

Never use a condom more than once.

Never blow up a condom before using it. If a condom tears, use a spermicide immediately. When in doubt, consult a physician for the morning-after pill. Store condoms in a cool place that is easily accessible.

7.5 Risk of transmission of HIV and STDs

	Activity	Risk of HIV	Risk of STD
1.	Sharing a razor	Slight	Moderate (hepatitis B & C)
2.	Caresses	None	None
3.	Massage	None	None
4.	Mutual masturbation	None (if no contact with mucosa, skin wound, and secretions)	Slight (herpes)
5.	Hugging while naked	None	None (except for crabs)
6.	Vulva–oral contact with protection (dental dam)	None	None
7.	Digital–anal penetration	None	Slight (intestinal parasites and hepatitis A)
8.	Kissing the other's body	None	None
9.	Nonsterilized needles for tattoo and body piercing	Moderate	Moderate (hepatitis B & C)
10.	Bathing with partner	None	None
11.	Rubbing of genitals	Slight	Moderate (genital warts, herpes, crabs)
12.	Oral–penile contact with condom	None	None
13.	Vaginal penetration with a condom	Slight	Slight (syphilis, genital warts, herpes, crabs)
14.	Anal–oral contact	Moderate	High (intestinal parasites, hepatitis A, genital warts, herpes)
15.	Receiving a vaccination	None	None
16.	HIV+ person coughing	None	None
17.	Being bitten by HIV+ person	Slight	Slight (hepatitis B & C)
18.	Touching an HIV+ person	None	None
19.	Kissing and exchanging saliva	Slight	Slight (herpes)
20.	Anal penetration with condom	Slight	Slight (syphilis, crabs, genital warts, herpes)
21.	Vaginal penetration	High	High
22.	Oral–vulva/oral–penile contact	Medium	Moderate (syphilis, hepatitis B, herpes)
23.	Abstinence	None	None
24.	Sharing needles	High	High
25.	Sharing sex toys	High	High
26.	Anal penetration	High	High
27.	Comforting someone who is crying	None	None
28.	Kissing on the cheek	None	None
29.	Solitary masturbation	None	None

Sexual orientation
(90 minutes)

General goals

To encourage the participants to talk about homosexuality in a positive manner in order to encourage the acceptance of differences. See 8.1, "Information for the group leader", for further discussion of this.

1. Hand out Worksheet 8.2, "Myths about sexual orientation" and begin the discussion by asking the participants to give their opinions about the statements (30 minutes).

2. Evaluate the degree of openness amongst participants in their attitudes to homosexuality. In order to do this, ask them to complete the quiz "Am I homophobic?" (Worksheet 8.3) (30 minutes).

3. Show a documentary on homosexuality or have a discussion around the prejudices and stereotypes that exist about sexual diversity (30 minutes).

Source material: Durocher, L. and Fortier, M. (1999) *Programme d'éducation sexuelle des Centres jeunesse de Montréal.*   153
Montréal: Le Centre jeunesse de Montréal – Institut Universitaire.

8.1 Information for the group leader

It is not easy to talk about sexual orientation with groups of adolescents. It should be noted with the group that having had a homosexual experience during adolescence does not necessarily mean that an individual has a homosexual orientation. Many individuals have, at some time or another, homosexual fantasies. Many boys and girls play sexual games with same-sex friends during childhood or adolescence. This does not necessarily mean that they are homosexual. However, sexual orientation often becomes defined during adolescence, after puberty.

The activities presented in this workshop allow participants to identify their values with respect to relationships and sexuality and facilitate discussion of these topics. The values that some people express may be different from your own. As leader, your attitude plays an important role in allowing the participants to express themselves. If you have moralistic attitudes and are judgemental, participants won't speak or may be challenging.

The subject of homosexuality can raise strong feelings. Some adolescents may have very blunt opinions and can make jokes which can be hurtful to others. You should consider the fact that some members of the group may be young gay men or lesbians who are in the process of questioning their sexual orientation. You must be ready to listen, without judging, to an adolescent who may be questioning his/her sexual orientation.

It is also important to use appropriate language and to know which words and expressions can be used (gay, lesbian, homosexual, bisexual) and which are laden with prejudice ("fag", "queen", "dyke", "butch", etc.).

In order to reduce any chance of ambiguity, we suggest that the term "partner" be used throughout the programme, instead of "boyfriend", "girlfriend", "spouse", or other. You should also tell the group that the word "couple" is as valid for two men or two women as it is for a man and a woman. This choice of language limits the danger of reinforcing stereotypes.

Goals of this workshop

The goal of this workshop is to encourage the participants to talk about homosexuality in a positive manner in order to encourage the acceptance of differences.

- Encourage participants to recognize and consider the differences and the opinions of others.

- Allow them to express their own points of view, regardless of what they are, by encouraging the group to listen and share.

- Allow each individual to identify their own values with respect to homosexuality, and to reflect upon and share these values.

154   Source material: Durocher, L. and Fortier, M. (1999) *Programme d'éducation sexuelle des Centres jeunesse de Montréal.* Montréal: Le Centre jeunesse de Montréal – Institut Universitaire.

- Lead participants to identify the prejudices and stereotypes that exist about homosexuality.

- Encourage a discussion on the consequences of homophobia.

- Bring the adolescents to a point where they can show increased comprehension and compassion towards others.

Source material: Durocher, L. and Fortier, M. (1999) *Programme d'éducation sexuelle des Centres jeunesse de Montréal.* 155
Montréal: Le Centre jeunesse de Montréal – Institut Universitaire.

✓

8.2 Myths about sexual orientation

An employer can fire an employee because he or she is homosexual

A homosexual couple cannot have children

A homosexual couple cannot raise children properly

In a homosexual couple, there is always a "guy" type and a "girl" type

All gay men are sex maniacs

All young people who have had a homosexual experience during adolescence are homosexuals

All gay men have AIDS

It's not normal to be homosexual

All lesbians are "tomboys"

Homosexual men and women have several sexual partners

If a homosexual person speaks to me, he/she is surely coming on to me

Homosexuality is a disease

Few adolescents ask themselves questions about their sexual orientation

8.3 Am I homophobic?

"Homophobia" consists of a series of negative attitudes towards homosexuality. It is manifested by insults, disparaging remarks, or physical violence.

Answering this questionnaire will allow you to stop and think about your values and your behaviours related to homosexuality. There are no right or wrong answers. Remember, no one is watching or judging you. Circle the answer that seems appropriate to you.

1 – Not at all   2 – Slightly   3 – Most of the time   4 – Always

1. I would be uncomfortable if I knew that someone of my gender found me attractive.

    1   2   3   4

2. I would be uncomfortable if I were attracted to someone of the same sex.

    1   2   3   4

3. I would be disappointed to learn that one of my friends was gay or lesbian.

    1   2   3   4

4. I would feel nervous in a group of homosexual individuals.

    1   2   3   4

5. I would feel disturbed if I knew that one of my teachers was homosexual.

    1   2   3   4

6. I would feel disgusted if I saw two men or two women kissing in the street.

    1   2   3   4

7. I would feel uncomfortable if my neighbour was homosexual.

    1   2   3   4

8. At a party, I would feel uncomfortable talking to someone who was gay or lesbian.

    1   2   3   4

9. I would feel uncomfortable consulting a gay or lesbian physician.

    1   2   3   4

10. I would feel uncomfortable crossing a mainly gay neighbourhood.

    1   2   3   4

✓

Results

10–20 points: You seem to have no trouble accepting homosexual individuals. Your attitudes and behaviours towards homosexual individuals are generally open-minded and relaxed. Your openness is very refreshing.

20–30 points: You are of two minds: you can accept the fact that homosexuality exists but have some reservations. You will have better contacts with people if you are a bit more accepting and if you allow yourself to open up more.

30–40 points: Homosexuality is difficult for you to accept. You have a hard time feeling comfortable with this reality. It might be helpful for you to reassess some of your relationships with gays and lesbians in your surroundings or elsewhere.

Alcohol, drugs, and sexuality
(90 minutes)

General goals

To enable participants to recognize and prevent the negative effects of drug and alcohol abuse on sexual pleasure and health. (see 9.1, "Information for the group leader", for further information.)

1. Discuss the relationship of alcohol and drugs to sexuality, and the different motivations for their use (10 minutes) (see Worksheet 9.2, "Discussion tips for group leaders").

2. Activity: "Scenario for an EXCITING sexual and romantic encounter" (Worksheet 9.3b).

    Explain the goal of the activity, (see 9.3a, "Best scenario: information for the group leader"). You can create a scenario through the use of collage or sketches according to the participants' preferences. Separate the group into two teams and ask them to fill out Worksheet 9.3b (40 minutes).

    The two teams should then present their results to the others (2 × 20 minutes per team – 40 minutes).

3. Those who would like to know more can undertake a personal reflection activity using Worksheet 9.4 (to be completed at home).

4. Distribute the brochure "Young People and Alcohol" found on *www.msss.gouv.qc.ca.*

Source material: Durocher, L. and Fortier, M. (1999) *Programme d'éducation sexuelle des Centres jeunesse de Montréal.* 159
Montréal: Le Centre jeunesse de Montréal – Institut Universitaire.

9.1 Information for the group leader

Why include a section on drugs and alcohol in a sexual education programme? A survey conducted by Health Quebec (Health Quebec, Government of Quebec 1991) on the sexual behaviours of 12- to 18-year-olds indicated that alcohol and drug use do have some influence on sexual behaviours in this age group. They found that those who were sexually active consumed twice as much alcohol and drugs as those who were not. Almost three quarters of the young people surveyed who did use alcohol and drugs, and over half of those who didn't, did not use a condom. Increased intoxication raised the likelihood of young people engaging in risky sexual behaviours. Young people should therefore be made aware of situations involving alcohol or drugs in which there may be an increased risk of them losing control, and must be encouraged to adopt attitudes that will lead to safe and responsible sexual behaviour.

The impact of drugs and alcohol on sexuality differs from one person to the next and depends on several factors: the type and quantity of substance used, the individual using it (personality, physical and psychological health), and the environment within which the individual finds him/herself (place, surroundings, cost of the substance, means used to obtain it). Drug and alcohol use may also impact upon the dynamics of sexual relations. Having sexual relations while under the influence of drugs or alcohol may be pleasurable for some, but for others it leads to a decrease in libido and sexual capacity. Those who abuse these substances may be at a greater risk of turning to prostitution to obtain drugs or pay for their drug habit.

It is important for you, as a group leader, to be as impartial as possible. Adopting a position based solely upon "zero tolerance" of drug and alcohol use is not helpful. Anti-alcohol and drug use propaganda is unrealistic and ineffective and can, paradoxically, incite some young people to use more. Adolescents are not going to view drugs and alcohol as problematic just because an overly-protective or moralistic tone is employed.

It is also important to avoid being categorical when dealing with the effects of drug and alcohol use. Someone in the group will inevitably claim to know people who have been using drugs and alcohol for a long time without any ill-effects. The discourse should therefore be focussed on *possible* risks. In order to facilitate a healthy discussion about alcohol and drugs, respect between adolescents and adults must be maintained, accurate and reasonable information must be conveyed, and a non-judgemental and non-moralistic tone must be favoured.

 Source material: Durocher, L. and Fortier, M. (1999) *Programme d'éducation sexuelle des Centres jeunesse de Montréal.* Montréal: Le Centre jeunesse de Montréal – Institut Universitaire.

Goals of this workshop

The goal of this workshop is to raise the participants' awareness of the potential negative impact of drug and alcohol abuse on their sexual health and pleasure.

- Identify the possible consequences of drug and alcohol use on sexual health.

- Identify the issues that should be considered when making decisions about whether or not to use drugs or alcohol.

- Discuss the reasons that might prompt young people to use drugs or alcohol.

- Allow the participants to think about and debunk certain myths about the magical effects of drugs and alcohol on sexuality.

- Reinforce safe attitudes and behaviours people should adopt when seeking rewarding sexual experiences.

- Provide an overview of the effects of using drugs and alcohol on individuals.

- Allow participants to identify the effects of using drugs or alcohol on sexual relations.

Source material: Durocher, L. and Fortier, M. (1999) *Programme d'éducation sexuelle des Centres jeunesse de Montréal.* 161 Montréal: Le Centre jeunesse de Montréal – Institut Universitaire.

9.2 Discussion tips for group leaders

Introduction to the topic

In order to facilitate a discussion on alcohol, drugs, and sexuality, we recommend that you start off with a brainstorming activity on the different reasons people might use them.

Ask the adolescents the following question and ask them to answer (a) off the top of their head (b) after thinking about it for a time.

Question: why do we use alcohol or drugs?

Allow the following reasons to come out (add any others):

- for pleasure or fun
- to be accepted by peers
- for excitement, because it's forbidden, sensation seeking
- to build identity, undergo a rite of passage
- to decrease anxiety, pain, sadness
- out of boredom, anger, joy, shyness
- to act out
- because of parental models
- because of personal experience

- to relax
- when you are at a party
- to stay awake
- to make you feel good
- to solve problems
- to forget
- to sleep
- to facilitate sexual relations
- to become more assertive
- because you are addicted
- to stimulate intellect or creativity.

Afterwards, ask the following questions in order to clarify the goals of the topic:

- What is the relationship between alcohol, drugs, and sex?
- Why do we talk about alcohol and drugs in a sexual education programme?

N.B. Answers can be found in Worksheet 9.1, "Information for the group leader".

 Source material: Durocher, L. and Fortier, M. (1999) *Programme d'éducation sexuelle des Centres jeunesse de Montréal.* Montréal: Le Centre jeunesse de Montréal – Institut Universitaire.

9.3a Best scenario: information for the group leader

Goals

1. Encourage participants to behave safely and responsibly in their quest for sexual pleasure.

2. Identify personal limits for alcohol or drugs in order to experience rewarding sexual contact.

Description

The teams of adolescents must come up with a scenario for an "exciting" sexual encounter. The scenario must be original, rewarding, respectful, and safe.

Material required

- Sheet and pencil for each team.

- Magazines, drawing or crafts materials.

- Cardboard, pencils, glue, scissors, etc.

- Contest sheet: one per team.

- Voting ballot sheet: one per participant.

Role of the group leader

Encourage participation and creativity. Encourage a positive exchange among the adolescents by reminding them to respect the opinions of others. Make sure participants respect the selection criteria of the contest (see Worksheet 9.3b). Ensure that the presentations go smoothly.

Steps

1. Explain to the group the nature of the activity and how it will unfold.

2. Ask them to think about and spontaneously note down all of the ideas about romantic relationships and their sexual ideals that come to mind.

3. Ask the participants to split into two groups to participate in a contest (distribute Worksheet 9.3b) and invite them to share amongst themselves the ideas that they have written down.

4. Ask each team to invent a scenario in which they have an exciting sexual experience that is original, rewarding, respectful, and safe.

Source material: Durocher, L. and Fortier, M. (1999) *Programme d'éducation sexuelle des Centres jeunesse de Montréal.* Montréal: Le Centre jeunesse de Montréal – Institut Universitaire.

5. Ask each team to present their scenario. This can be accomplished in various ways: drawings, or as a sketch or a reading of the scenario/script.

6. All the participants should discus the scenarios and vote for the winning scenario – that which they feel best fulfils the selection criteria.

7. To conclude the activity, have the participants talk about the fact that it is possible to have a very exciting sexual experience without using, or by limiting the use of, alcohol and drugs.

Questions for discussion around the different scenarios:

- Does this scenario represent a realistic situation?

- What is it that determines whether it is fun or pleasant?

- In the winning scenario, how do the partners feel and why?

 Source material: Durocher, L. and Fortier, M. (1999) *Programme d'éducation sexuelle des Centres jeunesse de Montréal.* Montréal: Le Centre jeunesse de Montréal – Institut Universitaire.

9.3b Scenario for an **EXCITING** sexual and romantic encounter

Selection criteria:

1. Originality.
2. Respect and sense of value.
3. Prevention of STDs and AIDS.
4. Pleasure.

This exercise is, first and foremost, about reflection. Its goal is to allow you to understand yourself better and to help you make and maintain your decisions in different situations.

In order to do this, imagine a situation…

Team name:

What are the circumstances? (party, date, romantic evening, vacation, etc.)

Describe the surroundings in which the intimate contact occurs.

✔

What happens, before, during, and after?

[blank box]

What are your sources of pleasure?

[blank box]

Prepare a short presentation to explain your scenario. You can use a poem, a sketch, a poster, a drawing, or you can simply read what you have written on this sheet.

9.4 The impact of using drugs and alcohol on my sexual behaviour and health

Look at the categories below and tick (✓) the statements that you agree with. Take a moment to think about the reasons why we use drugs or alcohol and the consequences that this may have on our sexual health.

Effects of drugs and alcohol

☐ Can decrease shyness.

☐ Removes our taboos.

☐ Can intensify our magical thinking (bad things only happen to others!).

☐ Can disturb the coordination of our movements, motor skills.

☐ Can create a physical or psychological dependency.

☐ Can create a pressing need for money.

☐ Other _____.

Consequences of using drugs and alcohol on my sexual behaviour

☐ Can help me make the first move.

☐ Can increase risky sexual behaviour, such as forgetting to use a condom.

☐ Can make it more difficult to use a condom properly.

☐ Can increase the possibility of turning to prostitution in order to obtain or finance the drugs or alcohol.

☐ Other _____.

Consequences of using drugs and alcohol on my sexual health

☐ Increases my risk of catching an STD, such as HIV.

☐ Increases the risk of unwanted pregnancy.

☐ Increases the likelihood of my experiencing physiological or psychological sexual problems (loss of desire, erection problems, etc.).

☐ Other _____.

WORKSHOP 10

Sexual abuse and inappropriate sexual behaviours
(90 minutes)

General goals

To familiarize the participants with the different forms of sexual abuse to which they may be exposed, be it within their family, outside of the family, or within their romantic relationships. The goal is to encourage young people to speak up for themselves in abusive situations and develop the means to protect themselves and others. This is discussed further in 10.1, "Information for the group leader".

1. Discuss privacy and its boundaries using Worksheet 10 2, "My privacy and its boundaries". Follow steps 1 to 3, provide examples, and underline the importance of privacy by explaining the difference between what is done in *private* and what is done in *public* (25 minutes).

2. What is sexual assault? Read Worksheet 10.3 with the group and discuss the ideas that are presented (20 minutes).

3. Ask the participants to judge the various situations presented in Worksheet 10.4 and to come back to the group to discuss their answers (30 minutes).

4. The group could watch the complementary video *No! How!!!* (Hingsburger, 1995a) which is specifically aimed at individuals with developmental disabilities. (10 minutes); see Diverse City Press at *www.diverse-city.com.*

Source material: Durocher, L. and Fortier, M. (1999) *Programme d'éducation sexuelle des Centres jeunesse de Montréal.* Montréal: Le Centre jeunesse de Montréal – Institut Universitaire.

10.1 Information for the group leader

These activities can sometimes provoke emotional reactions among participants, such as anger, sadness, or embarrassment, or they may provoke long silences. It is desirable for participants to feel that they can express themselves freely. Nonetheless, as group leader, you must focus on respect of the self and others by avoiding being judgemental. It may be necessary to remind the participants that we can condemn an act, but not a person. You may also experience strong emotional reactions yourself. These are normal and should be recognized, but must not be allowed to get in the way of the activity.

Discussions about sexual abuse may provoke acting out from some participants who might feel uncomfortable with the subject, or become impulsive when the discussion goes into more depth. It is therefore possible that, for a period of time, behaviours such as exhibitionism, voyeurism, touching, or similar may occur. These behaviours are to be expected and should in no way undermine the importance of this topic.

Activities dealing with sexual abuse may also trigger disclosures from participants. You must be ready to receive a disclosure of abuse and must ensure that the participant receives the necessary attention. You must reiterate, many times, the importance of identifying a trustworthy person to whom the participant may go, so that he/she does not remain trapped within the secret of sexual abuse. Nevertheless, you should avoid generating feelings of guilt in those who choose not to disclose or who continue to live with a secret. They may not feel ready to reveal their experiences or may not have previously realized that they were experiencing sexual abuse, either because of their age or their level of awareness. In addition, participants should understand that individuals who have been sexually abused are in no way responsible for the abuse.

It is important to explain that individuals who have experienced some form of sexual abuse can access the help that they and their families need. Youth centres offer services and programmes to help adolescents who have been sexually abused and to help those who themselves abuse. As group leader you must be well informed about the different services that exist. During this session, it is important that the participants hear that they can, with support, recover from these experiences. It is also important to avoid conveying the message that someone who has experienced sexual abuse will automatically become someone who abuses. Some participants could unfortunately come to the mistaken conclusion that they are inevitably destined to repeat these acts of abuse (Paquette *et al.*, 1995, cited in Durocher and Fortier, 1999).

Goals of this workshop

The goal of this workshop is to familiarize the participants with the different forms of sexual abuse to which they may be exposed, encourage participants to

Source material: Durocher, L. and Fortier, M. (1999) *Programme d'éducation sexuelle des Centres jeunesse de Montréal.* 169
Montréal: Le Centre jeunesse de Montréal – Institut Universitaire.

speak up in abusive situations and develop the means to protect themselves and others.

- Identify the different forms of sexual abuse that can be experienced by males and females in our society.

- Allow participants to identify their own boundaries regarding privacy and to clarify their notions of consent.

- Reflect upon the different forms of sexual abuse that can exist within the context of dating.

- Encourage participants to recognize the importance of confiding in someone if they are victims of sexual abuse and inform them of the resources and laws that can help them.

- Provide them with information about the resources and help that individuals who commit acts of sexual abuse can receive.

170   Source material: Durocher, L. and Fortier, M. (1999) *Programme d'éducation sexuelle des Centres jeunesse de Montréal.* Montréal: Le Centre jeunesse de Montréal – Institut Universitaire.

10.2 My privacy and its boundaries

1. To begin, present the goals of the activity and ask participants to describe briefly what privacy means to them.

2. Invite participants to name situations in which privacy is not respected. What activities are done in private? In public? To begin, provide examples where personal privacy can be threatened in the context of everyday life. Continue by providing examples of acts that could violate someone's privacy in intimate situations: entering someone's room without knocking, walking around in underwear without being concerned about the discomfort that this can prompt in others, going to the bathroom without closing the door, mocking a couple who are kissing, grabbing your girlfriend's breast in the presence of other people, forcing others to kiss you, etc.

3. In parallel, direct the discussion towards the importance of identifying one's own personal boundaries and of being clear about providing consent. Here are some suggestions of questions to ask:

   - Why is it important to set one's own boundaries?

   - How can we express our limits clearly?

   - Why is it sometimes difficult to have our limits respected?

   - Do you think that it is possible to forget to respect someone else's limits?

   - Do you recall situations where your limits were not respected? Why weren't they respected?

   - Can a person use alcohol as an excuse for having been abusive?

   - What does "giving consent" mean? How do we give our consent to someone?

   - In what ways might our romantic partner lack respect for our privacy?

4. To end the activity, review the main points about consent between two individuals and invite the participants to give tips and hints about different ways of clearly saying "no" to someone.

Source material: Durocher, L. and Fortier, M. (1999) *Programme d'éducation sexuelle des Centres jeunesse de Montréal.* 171
Montréal: Le Centre jeunesse de Montréal – Institut Universitaire.

✓

10.3 Stop sexual assault

What is sexual assault? It is...

- ...when a person tries to kiss you, touch you, and caress your genitals (fondling) without your permission.

- ...being forced to touch or caress the sexual parts of someone else (fondling).

- ...when someone wants or forces you to perform sexual acts on them when you do not want to.

- ...when someone forces you to have sexual relations with them.

- ...when a member of an individual's family, including parents, siblings or stepsiblings, grandparents, etc. has sexual relations with that individual. This is called "incest".

- ...being forced into committing sexual acts in front of other people.

- ...being forced to participate in sexual activities with animals.

Whether or not they use violence,
whether they are a stranger or someone you know:
when someone sexually assaults you they commit a crime.

It is worth remembering the following points:

- A person who sexually assaults someone doesn't always do it in the same way.

- Someone can sexually assault you using physical or verbal violence (threats) to make you do what they want. It is also possible for them to sexually assault you without using any form of violence at all.

- The sexual aggressor may abuse your trust to perform sexual acts on you or make you take part in sexual acts. He or she can also take advantage of the affection that you feel for him or her to perform sexual acts on you or make you take part in sexual acts. This is called "sexual abuse".

- The aggressor may be a stranger, someone you have seen before, or someone you know very well, even a member of your family.

10.4 Sexuality and the law: It's up to you to judge!

1. Julian and Sophie broke up three weeks ago. Julian has difficulty accepting the situation. He is constantly making anonymous phone calls to Sophie and checks all her comings and goings.
   - ☐ acceptable
   - ☐ tolerable
   - ☐ unacceptable

2. Mark demands that his girlfriend has sex with him, although she doesn't want to. He feels that she should because they've been going out for a while.
   - ☐ acceptable
   - ☐ tolerable
   - ☐ unacceptable

3. Mary is 13 years old. Her father occasionally asks her to engage in sexual activities with him. Her father is not violent with her; instead, he gives her everything she wants.
   - ☐ acceptable
   - ☐ tolerable
   - ☐ unacceptable

4. In the subway, a man frequently gets sexual pleasure by showing his penis.
   - ☐ acceptable
   - ☐ tolerable
   - ☐ unacceptable

5. Justine is 17 years old and has sexual relations with her 14-year-old boyfriend.
   - ☐ acceptable
   - ☐ tolerable
   - ☐ unacceptable

6. Sylvie works in a restaurant. Mike, the manager, finds her attractive, and threatens to fire her if she refuses to have sexual relations with him.
   - ☐ acceptable
   - ☐ tolerable
   - ☐ unacceptable

7. Fred regularly receives obscene phone calls.
   - ☐ acceptable
   - ☐ tolerable
   - ☐ unacceptable

8. Larry is 16 years old and is a monitor at a camp for 12- to 14-year-olds. As monitor, Larry is in a position of authority and trust with respect to the kids in his group. On several occasions, Larry has urged Naomi, a 14-year-old girl, to kiss him and touch his genitals.
   - ☐ acceptable
   - ☐ tolerable
   - ☐ unacceptable

WORKSHOP 11

Sexism and violence in romantic relationships
(90 minutes)

General goals

To alert participants to sexist and abusive behaviours and their consequences.

1. Discuss various kinds of social interactions: sexual intimacy, family and social relations etc. Complete the activity described in 11.1, "Social circles: information for the group leader" (adapted from Walker-Hirsch and Champagne, 1986) (30 minutes).

2. *Making Waves*: programme about sexual abuse in romantic relationships (40 minutes). See 11.2, "Making Waves: information for the group leader" for guidance.

3. Optional activity: Worksheet 11.3 can be completed by participants who are currently in a relationship (5–10 minutes).

174   Source material: Durocher, L. and Fortier, M. (1999) *Programme d'éducation sexuelle des Centres jeunesse de Montréal.*
Montréal: Le Centre jeunesse de Montréal – Institut Universitaire.

11.1 Social circles: information for the group leader

Draw three concentric circles on a large sheet or board where the smallest circle is green, the middle one is yellow, and the largest circle is red. The colours indicate when intimate behaviours are appropriate (green) or inappropriate (red), and with whom only certain kinds of intimate behaviour are appropriate (yellow).

- The *green* circle is the circle of intimacy.

- The *yellow* circle corresponds to family relationships.

- The *red* circle symbolizes social relationships.

First, ask participants to write on pieces of paper or card the names of partners, family members, friends and people within their environment such as shopkeepers, teachers, bus drivers. They should then place the pieces of paper in the circle that they think is most appropriate. On other pieces of paper they should write down different behaviours, for example "kissing on the lips", "saying hello", and they should then place these in the circles where they think they are most appropriate. The group leader should encourage the participants to say why they chose certain circles for certain people and behaviours. Then the group leader can start moving cards around. For example perhaps "being naked together" can be moved from the green circle to the yellow circle, and the group should discuss in which circumstances this is inappropriate and why. The group leader should always bear in mind the ages, experiences, and cultural backgrounds of the participants.

Below are some examples of what might be placed in each circle:

- A participant and his partner (if he has one) can be found in the green circle. Appropriate behaviours include: kissing on the lips, having an intimate or sexual contact, talking about feelings, sleeping together, getting undressed, respecting others' privacy, etc.

- The yellow circle might contain the name of a participant's mother or the name of a close friend. Appropriate behaviours include: kissing on the cheek, hugging, shaking hands, talking about feelings, etc. Inappropriate behaviours include: kissing on the lips, having an intimate or sexual contact, etc.

- In the red circle there might be the names of participants' classmates, teachers – even strangers in the street. Appropriate behaviours include: smiling, saying hello, shaking hands, not giving personal information, keeping an appropriate distance, etc. Inappropriate behaviours include: undressing, touching a private part, having a sexual contact, etc.

Adapted from Walker-Hirsch and Champagne (1986)

11.2 Making Waves: information for the group leader

Making Waves is a project that educates teenagers about sexual violence in relationships. It provides resources for teenagers, teachers and counsellors. Basic information is available for free at *www.mwaves.org/relationships.htm*. A student manual on dating violence and resource material for teachers and guidance counsellors can be purchased from Making Waves. Their activities target violence in romantic relationships. Exercises help participants to talk about violence and understand the cycle of violence.

Some of the topics covered in *Making Waves* are:

- Notions of context and space: private and public places.

- Limits of love (respectful and unhealthy situations, abusive relationships).

- What is violence in a romantic relationship?

- How to react when faced with a situation of sexual abuse.

- Sexuality and the law: judging different situations and exploring what is acceptable or not.

- Warning signs: how to detect if someone is being excessively jealous, explosive, depressed, agitated, or strange. How to prevent sexual abuse.

- How to help yourself or a friend recognize aggression.

The group leader should select those elements of the programme that are deemed appropriate for the group.

11.3 Me, abused in my romantic relationship?

A romantic relationship can occupy a huge part of our lives. Sometimes, without realizing it, we forget our own needs so that we can satisfy those of our partner. What influence does your partner have? Do you feel abused in your relationship? Answer the following questions and look at your score.

A – Never   B – Sometimes   C – Often

1. My partner says demeaning things about me.

   A   B   C

2. My partner discourages me from spending time alone with my friends.

   A   B   C

3. During sex, my partner insists that I engage in behaviours that I don't like.

   A   B   C

4. I force myself to have sexual relations to prove my love.

   A   B   C

5. My partner is the only one in our relationship who decides when we have sex.

   A   B   C

6. My partner says he/she is too busy to listen to me when I want to talk about our relationship.

   A   B   C

7. When my partner abuses alcohol or drugs I feel that he/she does not respect me.

   A   B   C

8. My partner makes hurtful or embarrassing sexual comments about me in the presence of friends.

   A   B   C

9. Our sexual relations bring me more fear than pleasure.

   A   B   C

10. My partner thinks that when I say NO it means YES.

    A   B   C

Results

Calculate your score:

1 point each time you choose A
2 points each time you choose B
3 points each time you choose C

Final score: _____

10–14 points: There doesn't seem to be any abuse between your partner and you in your relationship. Be in tune with what you feel and don't hesitate to say NO to anything you don't feel like doing.

15–23 points: There are some signs of abuse in your relationship. Abuse shouldn't have any place in your life. Have confidence in yourself, be direct when you feel abused and say NO when you don't feel like doing something. If you feel uncomfortable with a situation, ask someone you can trust for help. It is important to be in tune with what you feel.

24 or more points: Abusive relationships are neither healthy nor acceptable and should not tolerate the situation you are in. You need help. Don't hesitate to talk to someone you trust; this person will be able to help you. Everyone should be able to blossom in their relationship.

Managing emotions, theory of mind, and intimacy
(90 minutes)

General goals

To learn to decode the thoughts and feelings of others while fostering better communication skills among the participants.

1. Present the rationale behind the theory of mind-blindness. Explain why it is important to communicate our intentions and emotions appropriately to others if we are to have good interpersonal relationships (10 minutes).

2. If your group consists of young adolescents, begin with the mind-reading activities of Howlin *et al.* (1999) (15 minutes).

3. Cut up and hand out the different stories and emotions cards from Worksheet 12.1. Participants should act out the different emotions (nonverbally), with the rest of the group trying to identify the emotion or scenario that is being acted. If you have access to it, use the *Mind-reading* software (Baron-Cohen *et al.*, 2004) (60 minutes).

4. Optional activity: the group leader can help participants to write a Social Story™ as explained in *Writing Social Stories* (Gray, 2000) using the cards from Worksheet 12.1 as a starting point. The whole group can choose one scenario, or each participant chooses a scenario individually.

5. Ask adolescent participants to complete Worksheet 12.2 to measure the progress of each participant and discuss the results with them individually.

12.1 Role-playing cards

I find you attractive	I invite someone to the movies
I introduce myself	You have quite an effect on me
I'm nervous because I don't feel comfortable in this situation	I'm worried because I don't know this person well enough
My girlfriend/boyfriend hurt my feelings	I feel good when I spend time with you
My mind is at ease. I used contraceptives	I'm disappointed because my girlfriend/boyfriend doesn't agree to use contraception
I'm worried. I don't think that this person has good intentions	I have fun when I participate in an intimate activity
My heart pounds when I kiss you	I tremble with fear when a stranger invites me to his apartment
I feel comfortable because I know you well	I'm pleased with myself because I initiated a conversation
I'm happy because my girlfriend/boyfriend gave me a hug	I run away when I feel in danger
I can't take negative comments about my behaviour. I get carried away easily	I'm bad and aggressive because I feel alone and isolated

12.2 Adolescent questionnaire 2

Name: _____

Date: _____

Test your knowledge!   /10

1. Love between two people can only develop after having had sexual relations.
    ☐ true
    ☐ false

2. The foetus (unborn baby) is conceived by the joining of the _____ and the sperm.

    (a) uterus

    (b) penis

    ©) ovum

    (d) vagina

3. For there to be a sexual relation between two people, penetration of the penis into the vagina *must* occur.
    ☐ true
    ☐ false

4. If used correctly, the condom is the most effective means of preventing both pregnancy and the transmission of STDs.
    ☐ true
    ☐ false

5. In a homosexual couple, there is always one partner who has the role of "guy" and one partner who has the role of "girl".
    ☐ true
    ☐ false

6. Alcohol use makes sexual relations more pleasant.
    ☐ true
    ☐ false

7. A woman's role is to take care of the home and raise the children.
   ☐ true
   ☐ false

8. Physical beauty is the main ingredient in successful sexual behaviours.
   ☐ true
   ☐ false

9. Consent between two partners prevents sexual harassment or sexual abuse from taking place.
   ☐ true
   ☐ false

10. When I have an idea in my mind, other people have the same idea.
    ☐ true
    ☐ false

Appendix

The sexual profile of adults with Asperger's Syndrome: The need for support and intervention

Isabelle Hénault and Tony Attwood

Very little is known about the sexuality of individuals with AS. A study conducted in collaboration with Dr Tony Attwood began in 2001 with the aim of exploring the sexual profile of individuals with AS and addressing the following research question: "Do individuals diagnosed with AS present a sexual profile distinct from that of the general population?" The preliminary results of the study are presented and analysed in this Appendix. The study is still under way as we intend to involve a larger number of people and thus obtain a more complete picture of adult sexuality.

Participants in the study completed the Derogatis Sexual Function Inventory (DSFI; Derogatis and Melisaratos, 1982), a measure that provides a comprehensive assessment of behaviour, attitudes, sexual preference, and fantasy life of individuals and accumulates a maximum amount of information on sexuality. The inventory covers 11 aspects of sexuality, including desire, satisfaction and sexual values, for which general population norms have been established and which are measured on subscales. As the questionnaire explores sensitive topics, it was mailed to the 28 participants in Canada, Australia, the USA, and France, and completed anonymously.

There are a number of obstacles to exploring the sexual universe of individuals with AS: there is a lack of research and available data in this field, and the lack of sociosexual skills in AS individuals often increases their resistance to and misunderstanding of sexual relationships, and, indeed, the likelihood of their behaviour being misunderstood by others.

The results suggest that individuals with AS have levels of sexual interest that are comparable to those of the general population. On the other hand, the communication difficulties that they experience, combined with their lack of social skills, serve to increase the likelihood that they will experience symptoms of depression and may display inappropriate sociosexual behaviours.

Study

Participants

A total of 28 adults (19 men and 9 women) participated in the study and anonymously completed the DSFI, which they received by mail. Three transsexuals with AS (one man and two women) agreed to participate in the study. The mean age of the participants was 34 years, ranging from 18 to 64 years. Twenty-one participants had either received a formal diagnosis of AS or achieved a score above a critical level of 32 on the Autism Spectrum Quotient (AQ; Baron-Cohen *et al.*, 2001). The AQ measures the extent of autistic traits in adults of normal intelligence. Five participants had been diagnosed with high functioning autism and two had received a more general diagnosis of PDD. Characteristics and symptoms corresponded to diagnostic criteria for AS as defined in the *Diagnostic Statistical Manual of Mental Disorders* (DSM-IV; APA, 1994). Fourteen participants were residents of Canada, nine of Australia, three of the USA, and two of France. Sixteen were single and 12 were in relationships.

The DSFI

This self-report measure is subdivided into 11 subscales (information, experience, desire, attitudes, symptoms, affect, gender identity, fantasies, body image, satisfaction, and general sexual satisfaction). In order to establish the sexual profile of individuals with AS, scores and standard deviations obtained on each subscale were compared to those obtained from men and women in the general population. Some subscales of the DSFI are drawn from the Brief Symptom Inventory (BSI; Derogatis, 1975, in Derogatis and Melisaratos, 1982), which measures psychopathology. The Positive Symptom Distress Index (PSDI) and the General Severity Index (GSI) also influenced the design of the DSFI.

Results

Responses to each of the 11 subscales were compiled so that mean scores could be obtained. These were then compared to a population mean score of 50 (Derogatis and Melisaratos, 1982), making it possible to examine the distinct sexual profile of participants with AS. The results are presented in Table A.1 and Figure A.1.

The scores of the AS participants on four subscales (2, 5, 6 and 9 – experience, symptoms, affect, and body image) were situated two standard deviations below the general population norms. This represents a significant difference.

Table A.1 Mean scores and standard deviations obtained on subscales of the DSFI. Source: Hénault and Attwood (2004)

Subscales	M (n = 28)	SD	MM (n = 19)	SD	MF (n = 9)	SD
1. Information	40	15	39	12	43	18
2. Experience	36	11	34	11	38	12
3. Desire	42	11	43	10	40	13
4. Attitudes	44	13	44	14	44	11
5. Symptoms	37	10	37	9	37	12
6. Affect	38	13	37	14	38	11
7. Sexual roles	49	14	45	14	58	8
8. Fantasies	49	13	48	15	49	7
9. Body image	34	12	32	8	37	18
10. Satisfaction	40	10	41	8	38	14
11. General satisfaction	46	12	48	12	38	11

Key:
M = Mean scores
MM = Male mean scores
MF = Female mean scores
SD = Standard deviation
n = Number of participants

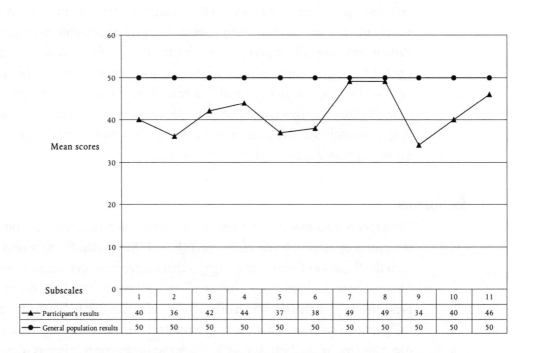

Figure A.1 Sexual profile of adults with Asperger's Syndrome. Source: Hénault and Attwood (2004)

Body image

The lowest mean score was found on the subscale for body image (M = 34, SD = 12). Respondents are asked to rate how satisfied they are with their body and whether they perceive it as attractive or desirable. The first section of the questionnaire addresses both genders and respondents are asked to rate statements such as "I am less attractive than I would like to be", "There are parts of my body I don't like at all", and "I would be embarrassed to be seen nude by a partner". The second section is divided by gender. Statements to be rated by men include "I have a well-proportioned body", "I am satisfied with the size of my penis", and "Women would find my body attractive"; for women they include "I am well built and well proportioned", "I have attractive breasts and attractive legs", and "Men would find my body attractive".

The results reveal that individuals with AS have a poor body image, which could lead to a low frequency of sexual activity. The more negative the body image, the fewer attempts by individuals to establish an intimate relationship with a partner. Such results contradict the hypothesis that individuals with AS or high functioning autism have little interest in the image that they project or few aesthetic concerns: on the contrary, they appeared quite aware of and sensitive to their body image, which they perceived negatively. Women's mean scores (M = 37, SD = 18) were higher than those of men (M = 32, SD = 8, in fact the lowest score observed on any of the subscales), which suggests that women have a slightly more positive body image than men and take an interest in their physical appearance and feminine image. Nonetheless, their result remains poor compared to the score of women in the general population.

Experiences

The experience subscale received the second lowest overall mean score for the AS participants (M = 36, SD = 11), based on a mean for the general population of 50. The DSFI asks participants to report on their experiences in the previous two months of a variety of activities, such as kissing, caressing genitals, masturbation, and intercourse. Participants generally experienced their first feeling of sexual desire at puberty (mean age = 14 years), but only started to have sexual experiences in their twenties. The mean age for the first experience involving intercourse was 22 years. Eleven participants were virgins; their ages ranged between 18 and 40 years; three women and eight men. Proportionately speaking, women in the study had more sexual experiences (M = 38, SD = 12) than did men (M = 34, SD = 11).

Symptoms

Participants also reported a substantial number of psychological and physiological symptoms of varying levels of distress (M = 37, SD = 10). These results are consistent with the findings of others that suggest that anxiety and depressed mood are found in 65% of individuals with AS (Sofronoff and Attwood, 2002). A list of 53 items was presented to participants who had to tick the symptoms that they had experienced over the past two weeks. Agitation, nervousness, loneliness, anxiety, fear, problems with digestion, insomnia, heat flushes, and guilt were terms participants selected as describing their general state. No gender differences were observed the scores for women were M = 37, SD = 12; for men, M = 37, SD= 9.

Affect

The affect scale yielded the fourth lowest score from the participants with AS (M = 38, SD = 10). Anxiety and sadness were the predominant emotions reported by participants. Emotions such as "unhappy", "tense", and "bitter" were reported more frequently than "energetic", "joyful", or "happy". Participants also had to rate their emotions according to five qualifiers: never, rarely, sometimes, frequently, and always. In general, the intensity of the emotions was rated at the extreme poles; that is, participants usually reported "never", "frequently", or "always". Very few emotions were experienced "rarely" or "sometimes". This way of experiencing and managing emotion is quite typical of individuals with AS. They have a rigid conception of emotion: emotions such as joy, anger, and sadness were found to be part of their repertoire, but more subtle feelings, such as amicability, fulfilment, shame, or spite, were rarely reported. Results on the affect subscale revealed that participants tended to experience more negative emotions than the general population. This is directly related to the low self-esteem and psychological and physiological symptoms reported. Negative affect leads to solitude and isolation. The mean score for men (M = 37, SD = 14) was only slightly lower than that obtained for women (M = 38, SD = 11), which leads us to conclude that they effectively share the same emotions.

Information

The information subscale was one of the five that produced mean scores between 40 and 49 (one standard deviation below the mean for the general population). The information subscale assesses general knowledge about sexuality. Participants had to answer true or false to 26 statements about sexuality, for example "A woman who has had a hysterectomy can no longer experience orgasm", "Most men and women lose interest in sex after age 60", and "Erection in the male is brought about by congestion of blood in the penis". The overall mean score (M = 40, SD = 15) confirms the hypothesis that individuals with AS and high functioning autism have a below average level of sexual knowledge, although women (M = 43, SD = 18) knew more about sexuality than men (M = 39, SD = 12).

Given their thirst for knowledge and high levels of curiosity, it is quite surprising that individuals with AS did not score higher. The participants lacked information on physiology, behaviour, and sexual health, and their sexual knowledge was based on common assumptions, possibly because of their limited sexual experience and the fact that most of them had never attended any sexual education classes. The majority of the information they possessed had been obtained through the media or other sources that were not always reliable. This lack of existing knowledge, and the twin motivations of curiosity and desire to find out more about sexuality, partly explain why interest in the sociosexual education programme is so high.

Satisfaction

Scores on the satisfaction subscale were similar to those found on the information subscale (M = 41, SD = 10). Ten statements in the questionnaire were used to determine participants' level of satisfaction and these included "There is not enough variety in my sex life", "Foreplay before intercourse is usually very arousing for me",

"Often I worry about my sexual performance", etc. Despite their limited sexual experiences, negative affect, and symptoms of agitation, anxiety, etc., male participants in the study were more satisfied with their sexual lives (M = 41, SD = 8) than the females (M = 38, SD = 14).

Desire

An interesting mean was obtained on the desire subscale (M = 42, SD = 11). This section of the DSFI includes the actual frequency of sexual behaviour (with and without a partner), what individuals perceive should be the ideal frequency, and sexual fantasies. It is divided into seven sections: frequency of sexual relations, masturbation, caresses, sexual fantasies, ideal frequency of sexual contact (as opposed to the real frequency), age of first sexual desire, and age of first intercourse. Despite their limited sexual experiences and the low frequency of their sexual activity, participants had a high level of desire. Desire was present but opportunities were rare, especially for those participants who were single. In general, the men had more sexual desire (M = 43, SD = 10) than the women (M = 40, SD = 13).

Attitudes

The mean score on the attitude subscale was 44 (SD = 13) and in general the participants' attitude towards sexuality was positive. In this section, using a five-point Likert scale (–2 "strongly disagree" to 2 "strongly agree") participants give their opinions about 30 statements, including "Premarital intercourse is beneficial to later marital adjustment", "Homosexuality is perverse and unhealthy", "Human genitals are somewhat disgusting to look at", and "Masturbation fantasies are healthy forms of sexual release". In general, the participants' lack of moral judgement left room for more liberal values, leading to open-mindedness around sexual diversity (homosexuality, bisexuality, or premarital relations). No gender differences were noted (for men, M = 44, SD = 14; for women, M = 44, SD = 11).

General satisfaction

The mean of the general satisfaction (GS) subscale was high (M = 46, SD = 12), considering the few sexual experiences and negative body image of the participants. To assess GS, participants had to evaluate their affective and sexual life on a scale of 0 ("could not be worse") to 8 ("could not be better"). Despite the high overall score, several discrepancies were noted. Twelve participants rated their sexual life as very bad or mediocre. Only four participants were very satisfied. Those remaining considered their sexual life to be acceptable. Globally, the overall mean resembled that of the general population. However, an important difference between men (M = 48, SD = 12) and women (M = 38, SD = 11) was observed. Women were clearly less satisfied about the frequency of their sexual life and the quality of their sexual relations. They wished for more diversity and general satisfaction. In contrast, men were more satisfied with their sexual life even if their frequency of sexual contact was limited. They felt that their sexual life was acceptable.

Fantasies

Participants seemed to have rich and diversified fantasy life. The mean of all participants was 49 ($\underline{SD}$ = 13); thus the number of their sexual fantasies resembled that of the general population ($\underline{M}$ = 50), which supports the hypothesis that individuals with AS have a fantasy life. The richness of images and scenarios evoked confirmed that the dimensions of desire and sexual imagery in this group were strongly developed. Approximately 20 different imaginary scenarios were presented in the questionnaire for participants to comment on: "Dressing in erotic garments", "Homosexual fantasies", "Oral–genital sex", "Mate-swapping fantasies". The most commonly reported fantasies were homosexual fantasies, intercourse, having more than one partner at once, wearing erotic clothing, and engaging in sexual acts. Men ($\underline{M}$ = 48, $\underline{SD}$ = 15) and women ($\underline{M}$ = 49, $\underline{SD}$ = 7) essentially reported the same number of fantasies. The nature and the content differed from one individual to the next, but in general the fantasies involved the presence of a sexual partner.

Sexual roles

Finally, the subscale measuring sexual roles obtained the same overall mean among participants as the fantasies subscale ($\underline{M}$ = 49, $\underline{SD}$ = 14). In general, participants in the study tended to attribute to themselves the personality traits associated with their gender. Males defined themselves as being definite, practical, logical, independent, routine-minded, and authoritarian. These characteristics are similar to those commonly associated with AS. Women characterized themselves as being sensitive, reserved, and gentle. Participants seemed to have a clear idea of what constituted their sexual role and were comfortable with their sexual roles and accompanying characteristics. In conclusion, the sense of belonging and gender identity (the sense of being male or female) seemed deeply rooted in their personalities. Men's mean scores ($\underline{M}$ = 45, $\underline{SD}$ = 14) were nevertheless lower than women's ($\underline{M}$ = 58, $\underline{SD}$ = 8), which was eight points higher than population norms. This would seem to indicate that the female participants readily perceived themselves as feminine.

Discussion

Negative body image, lack of sexual experiences, and symptoms of depression and anxiety contribute to the sexual dysfunctions observed in some individuals with AS. Lack of opportunities and a restrictive environment also increase the incidence of inappropriate sexual conduct.

The mean scores on the subscale for sexual desire, roles, and fantasies were all significant. These results confirm the hypothesis that individuals with high functioning autism and AS have sexual desires and a fantasy life comparable to those in the general population. In addition they appear to be quite comfortable with their respective social roles. The high frequency of the occurrence of their sexual desires may indicate that individuals with AS have a rich fantasy life. The results obtained on the fantasies and sexual roles subscales show that, in general, the AS sexual profile differs in several respects from that of the general population. Homosexual fantasies were mentioned several times. While there isn't necessarily any correlation between fantasy and behaviour since fantasies describe sexual preferences, not behaviour, sexual fantasies sometimes provide information about sexual orientation. Therefore although the incidence of homosexuality in the AS population remains unknown, we suspect that it is higher than in the general population.

Social norms do not seem to have much influence on body image, the sense of belonging to one's sex, and the erotic imagination of individuals with AS. They appear to act according to their internal desires regardless of whether these are directed to a person of the same or the opposite sex. One of the authors has recently been in contact with a discussion group composed of transgendered individuals with AS. Could there be a high comorbidity rate between PDDs and gender identity disorders? This hypothesis needs empirical research and we will continue to examine it in the context of this ongoing study; Chapter 4 of this book explores the notions of gender identity and sexual diversity in individuals with AS further.

Satisfaction can exist despite a low frequency of sexual intercourse, which may not be a problem for the person with AS – though it may be a problem for his or her partner. Some participants had only had one or two experiences of sexual intercourse in their lifetimes and they seemed fine about this. However, those who were still virgins were very concerned that they might remain so, especially in light of their limited social contacts, which caused them frustration and depression.

In general, the principal hypothesis was confirmed: individuals with AS have sexual desires and needs comparable to those of the general population. Their attitudes towards sexuality are positive, they have a rich fantasy life, but they lack sexual experience and their negative affect impacts on social and sexual interactions. One participant said that "Situations with lovers are quite delicate. It's as if my solitude and lack of sexual experience is visible. Many look at me and laugh…how can I help but feel inferior and unhappy?"

The results of this study confirm the importance of teaching social and sexual skills to individuals living with high functioning autism and AS (Haracopos and Pedersen, 1999). As suggested in the literature (Chipouras et al., 1982; Griffiths et al., 1989; Hellemans, 1996), a structured education programme designed to meet the needs of this population must be part of the services offered to them. The National Information Center for Children and Youth with Disabilities (1992), Kempton (1993), and Hingsburger (1993) all state that the more individuals are educated about sexuality, the more able they are to make informed and autonomous choices. This not only decreases the risk of sexual abuse, it allows individuals with autism access to a rewarding social and sexual life. Long-term consequences of the sociosexual skills training programme include improved self-esteem and this could counterbalance the negative body image reported on the DSFI questionnaires. The development of social skills decreases an individual's isolation and depression by creating an openness towards others, increasing interpersonal exchanges, and helping them to develop friendships and intimate relationships.

Further analyses

Additional information related to the personal histories of the participants showed that despite the lack of experience they had reported on the DSFI questionnaires, 43% of the participants were in a relationship and therefore had more general sexual experiences which allowed them to refine their knowledge, social skills, and capacity for intimacy. All participants had had experience of interpersonal relationships (with their parents, friends, partners, colleagues, classmates, etc.) and showed an interest in developing the skills needed to forge friendships and intimate relationships with the people in their environment.

Although all developed an interest in sexuality around the age of 14 years, 11 of the 28 participants were still virgins. They were also among the 16 single participants who were more dissatisfied with their emotional and sexual life ($M = 41$, $SD = 12$) than those who were in a relationship ($M = 52$, $SD = 11$). Diversity of sexual activities, frequency, and pleasure were also higher in the latter group.

The three transsexual participants obtained interesting scores on the subscales for attitude, image, and sexual roles. Of course, it is impossible to generalize on the basis of such a small sample; however, it may be helpful for understanding the variations within the AS population. The mean scores of the transsexuals on the attitude subscale were much higher ($M = 53$, $SD = 4$) than in the rest of the sample ($M = 35$, $SD = 13$). Their body image scores were lower than those obtained for the general population, and they were not entirely satisfied with the results of the hormonal and surgical interventions they had undergone, especially the appearance of the genitals. Their means scores on the roles subscale ($M = 52$, $SD = 18$) were also lower than those of the other partici-pants ($M = 49$, $SD = 14$). Their responses not only corresponded to the characteristics related to their biological sex, but to both sexes. They readily described themselves as having both masculine and feminine characteristics. This result indicates more flexibility than was observed in the other participants.

The need for education and support

By definition, individuals with AS are different from others. They have a different profile of social, cognitive, and communication abilities. They also have different life experiences. As a group, it is clear that their sexual desire is within the normal range but they have a poor body image, mediocre knowledge regarding sexuality, and relatively limited experience in intimate relationships. As a compensatory mechanism they may develop a fantasy life, but while this can trigger desire and sexual drive, individuals with AS should be encouraged to establish social relationships and a sexual life with real-life partners – not just in imaginary scenarios. Their different concept of social conventions can also lead to a greater degree of sexual diversity among them than among the general population. A lack of success with intimate relationships can contribute to an individual with AS developing depression or an anxiety disorder. Aspies are vulnerable to misinformation and misinterpretation, have difficulty commu-nicating thoughts and feelings, and often have tactile sensitivities that render some intimate activities physically uncomfortable.

Individuals with AS need understanding and support from their partners, families, friends, and relationship counselling agencies. The support should take the forms of attitude and advice. The remedial programmes on social cognition, particu-larly in the areas of friendship skills and empathy, that begin in the person's early childhood, should continue as they mature to include information and guidance on puberty, dating, sexual knowledge and identity, and intimacy. The goal is to provide people with AS with greater knowledge and more positive experiences so that their decision-making and self-esteem are improved. The programmes must accommodate the person's circumstances and the cognitive profile associated with AS. We are currently developing and evaluating individual, couple, and group therapy programmes on sexuality and relationships for adolescents and adults with AS.

This Appendix describes the preliminary results of an ongoing study using the Derogatis Sexual Functioning Inventory (DSFI) that will eventually include a sufficient number of subjects for a more detailed and robust statistical analysis. Nevertheless, a distinct pattern has been detected with adults who have AS and high functioning autism that warrants further empirical examination and the development of educational and counselling programmes based on their unusual profile of sexual knowledge and behaviour.

References, further reading, and resources

Abelson, A.G. (1981) "The development of gender identity in the autistic child." *Child: Care Health and Development 7*, 343–56.

Adolphs, R., Sears, L. and Piven, J. (2001) "Abnormal processing of social information from faces in autism." *Journal of Cognitive Neuroscience 13*, 2, 232–40.

Alarie, P. and Villeneuve, R. (1992) *L'impuissance: Évaluations et Solutions.* Montréal: Editions de l'Homme.

Aman, M.G., Richmond, G., Stewart, A.W., Bell, J.C. and Kissel, R.C. (1987) "The Aberrant Behavior Checklist: Factor structure and the effect of subject variables in American and New Zealand facilities." *American Journal of Mental Deficiency 91*, 570–8.

Aman, M.G. and Singh, N.N. (1986) *Aberrant Behavior Checklist: Manual.* East Aurora, NY: Slosson Educational Publications.

American Academy of Pediatrics (1996) "Sexuality education of children and adolescents with developmental disabilities." (RE9603) *Pediatrics 97*, 275–8.

APA (American Psychiatric Association) (1994) *Diagnostic and Statistical Manual of Mental Disorders, Fourth Edition* (DSM-IV). Washington, DC: APA.

Aquilla, P. (2003) "Sensory issues in individuals with Asperger Syndrome." *The Second National Conference on Asperger's Syndrome.* Toronto: Aspergers Society of Ontario.

Arturo Silva, J., Ferrari, M. and Leong, G. (2002) "The case of Jeffrey Dahmer: Sexual serial homicide from a neuropsychiatric developmental perspective." *Journal of Forensic Science 47*, 6, 1347–59.

Asperger, H. (1944) *Die "Autistischen Psychopathen" im Kindesalter. Les Psychopathes Autistiques pendant l'Enfance.* Translated into French in 1994 and published by Le Cannet: EDI Formation.

Asperweb France (2000) "Définition, historique et caractéristiques du syndrome d'Asperger." *http://perso.wanadoo.fr/asperweb*

Aston, M.C. (2001) *The Other Half of Asperger Syndrome.* London: The National Autistic Society.

Aston, M.C. (2003) *Aspergers in Love.* London: Jessica Kingsley Publishers.

Attwood, T. (1998a) *Asperger's Syndrome: A Guide for Parents and Professionals.* London: Jessica Kingsley Publishers.

Attwood, T. (1998b) "The links between social stories, comic strip conversations and the cognitive models of autism and Asperger's Syndrome." *The Morning News,* January, 3–6.

Attwood, T. (1999a) "Understanding and helping adolescents with Asperger's Syndrome." Conference for the Société Québécoise de l'Autisme, Montréal.

Attwood, T. (1999b) "Cognitive behaviour therapy to accommodate the cognitive profile of people with Asperger's Syndrome." *www.tonyattwood.com.au*

Attwood, T. (2000) "Strategies for improving the social integration of children with Asperger Syndrome." *Autism 4*, 85–104.

Attwood, T. (2002) Personal communication. Unpublished.

Attwood, T. (2003a) "Cognitive behaviour therapy." In L. Holliday Willey (ed.) *Asperger Syndrome in Adolescence: Living with the Ups, the Downs, and Things In Between.* London: Jessica Kingsley Publishers.

Attwood, T. (2003b) Lecture at the Third FAAAS International Conference. *www.faaas.org.*

Attwood, T. (2003c) "Indices of Friendship Observation Schedule." *www.tonyattwood.com.au*

Attwood, T. (2004a) *Exploring Feelings: Cognitive Behaviour Therapy to Manage Anger.* Arlington, TX: Future Horizons.

Attwood, T. (2004b) *Exploring Feelings: Cognitive Behaviour Therapy to Manage Anxiety.* Arlington, TX: Future Horizons.

Attwood, T. and Gray, C. (1999a) "Understanding and teaching friendship skills." *www.tonyattwood.com.au*

Attwood, T. and Gray, C. (1999b) "The discovery of 'Aspie' criteria." *The Morning News, 11,* 3. pp.1–7. *www.tonyattwood.com.au*

Barbach, L. (1997) *Loving Together: Sexual Enrichment Program.* New York: Brunner/Mazel.

Baron-Cohen, S., Wheelright, S., Skinner, R., Martin, J. and Clubley, E. (2001) "The Autism-Spectrum Quotient (AQ): Evidence from Asperger Syndrome/High functioning autism, males and females, scientists and mathematicians." *Journal of Autism and Developmental Disorders 31,* 1, 5–17.

Baron-Cohen, S., Golan, O., Wheelright, S. and Hill, J.J. (2004) *Mind-Reading: The Interactive Guide to Emotions.* Cambridge: Human Emotions.

Basso, M.J. (1997) *The Underground Guide to Teenage Sexuality.* Minneapolis, MN: Fairview Press.

Beaudoin, L., Bruneau, S., Ouellet, D., and Simard, R. (1980) *Ça ne peut plus durer.* Cliniques des jeunes St-Denis. Montréal: Bureau de Consultation Jeunesse Inc.

Bernier, S. and Lamy, M. (1998) *Programme d'entraînement aux habiletés sociales adapté pour une clientèle présentant un trouble envahissant du développement.* Hôpital Rivière-des-Prairies: Clinique des Troubles Envahissants du Développement.

Binet, A. (1887) "Le fétichisme dans l'amour." *Revue Philosophique 24,* 143–67; 252–74.

Boisvert, J.M. and Beaudry, M. (1979) *S'affirmer et communiquer.* Montréal: Éditions de l'Homme.

Boisvert, J.M. and Beaudry, M. (1985) *Principes de la communication.* Montréal: Hôpital Louis-H. Lafontaine.

Bouchard, P., Keller, Y. and Saint-Jean, N. (1988) *Dans les coulisses de l'intimité sexuelle.* Montréal: Fondation Jeunesse.

Bradley, S.J. and Zucker, K.J. (1997) "Gender identity disorder: A review of the past 10 years." *Journal of the American Academy of Child and Adolescent Psychiatry 36,* 872–80.

Brent, E., Rios, P., Happé, F. and Charman, T. (2001) "Performance of Children with Autism Spectrum Disorder on advance Theory of Mind tasks." *Autism 8,* 3, 283–299.

Calgary Birth Control Association (2002) *Counseling and Education. www.cbca.ab.ca*

Canadian Pharmaceutical Association (1994). *www.autisme.QC.ca*

Carnes, P. (1989) *Contrary to Love: Helping the Sexual Addict.* Minneapolis, MN: CompCare Publishers.

Carnes, P. (1993) *S'affranchir du secret: Sexualité compulsive.* Minneapolis, MN: CompCare Publishers.

Channon, S., Charman, T., Heap, J., Crawford, S. and Rios, P. (2001) "Real-life problem-solving in Asperger's Syndrome." *Journal of Autism and Development Disorders 31,* 461–9.

Chipouras, S., Cornelius, D., Daniels, F. and Makas, E. (1982) *Who Cares? A Handbook on Sex Education and Counseling Services for Disabled People.* Baltimore, MD: University Park Press.

Cohen, J. (1999) *The Penis Book.* New York: Fresh Ideas Daily.

Cohen-Kettenis, P.T. (2003) "Demographic characteristics, social competence, and behavior problems in children with gender identity disorders: A cross-national, cross-clinic comparative analysis." *Journal of Abnormal Child Psychology 1*, 41–53.

Coleman, E. (1991) "Compulsive sexual behavior: New concepts and treatments." *Journal of Psychology and Human Sexuality 4*, 37–52.

Cooper, S.A., Mohamed, W.N. and Collacott, R.A. (1993) "Possible Asperger's syndrome in a mentally handicapped transvestite offender." *Journal of Intellectual Disability Research 37*, 189–94.

Curnoe, S. and Langevin, R. (2002) "Personality and deviant sexual fantasies: An examination of the MMPIs of sex offenders." *Journal of Clinical Psychology 58*, 803–15.

De Myer, M.K. (1979) *Parents and Children in Autism.* London: John Wiley.

Debbaudt, D. (2001) *Autism, Advocates, and Law Enforcement Professionals: Recognizing and Reducing Risk Situations for People with Autism Spectrum Disorders.* London: Jessica Kingsley Publishers.

Debbaudt, D. (2002) *Avoiding Unfortunate Situations: A Collection of Experiences, Tips and Information from and about People with Autism and Other Developmental Disabilities and Their Encounters with Law Enforcement Agencies.* Detroit, MI: Wayne County Society for Autistic Citizens.

Département de Sexologie (1996) *Lexique des Termes Sexologiques.* Montréal: Université du Québec à Montréal.

Derogatis, L.R. and Melisaratos, N. (1982) *Inventaire du Fonctionnement Sexuel.* Baltimore, MD: Clinical Psychometric Research, Inc. *www.derogatis-tests.com*

Desaulniers, M.P. (2001) *Programme d'Éducation à la Vie Affective, Amoureuse et Sexuelle.* Trois-Rivières: Centre de services en déficience intellectuelle de la Mauricie et du Centre-du-Québec.

Dodson, B. (1974) *Liberating Masturbation.* New York: Three Rivers Press.

Dodson, B. (1996) *Sex for One: The Joy of Selfloving.* New York: Three Rivers Press.

Dorais, M. (1999) *Éloge de la diversité sexuelle.* Montréal: VLB Éditeurs.

Dubé, L. (1994) "Les relations interpersonnelles." In R.J. Vallerand (ed.) *Les fondements de la psychologie sociale.* Boucherville: Gaétan Morin.

Durocher, L. and Fortier, M. (1999) *Programme d'éducation sexuelle des Centres jeunesse de Montréal.* Montréal: Le Centre Jeunesse de Montréal – Institut Universitaire. Direction de la santé publique.

Ehlers, S. and Gillberg, C. (1993) "The epidemiology of Asperger syndrome: A total population study." *Journal of Child Psychology and Psychiatry 34*, 1327–50.

Erickson, E.H. (1963) *Childhood and Society* (second edition). New York: Norton.

Family Planning Queensland (2001) *Sexual and Reproductive Health.* Brisbane: Family Planning Queensland.

Ford, A. (1987) "Sex education for individuals with autism: Structuring information and opportunities." In D.J. Cohen, A.M. Donnellan and R. Paul (eds) *Handbook of Autism and Pervasive Developmental Disorders.* Maryland, MD: Winston.

Foreman, J. (2003) "A look at empathy, please!" Boston: Globe Newspaper Company. *www.boston.com/globe*

Fortin, N. and Thériault, J. (1995) "Intimité et satisfaction sexuelle." *Revue Sexologique 3*, 1, 37–58.

Frith, U. (1991) *Autism and Asperger Syndrome.* Cambridge: Cambridge University Press.

Gale, T. (2001) *Gale Encyclopaedia of Psychology.* Farmington Hills, MI: Gale Group.

Gallucci, G., Hackerman, F. and Schmidt, W. (2005) "Gender Identity Disorder in an Adult Male with Asperger's Syndrome." *Sexuality and Disability, 23*, 1, pp.35–40.

Ghaziuddin, M. and Tsai, L. (1991) "Brief report: Violence in Asperger syndrome; a critique." *Journal of Autism and Developmental Disorders 21*, 349–54.

Gillberg, C. (1983) "Éveil de la conscience sexuelle chez l'adolescent autistique." *L'avenir des autistes et psychotiques à travers différentes approches.* Paris: Actes du Congrès de Paris.

Gillberg, C. and Gillberg, C. (1989) "Asperger's syndrome – some epidemiological considerations: A research note." *Journal of Child Psychology and Psychiatry 30,* 631–8.

Gilliam, J.E. (2001) *Gilliam Asperger's Disorder Scale.* Kingsland, TX: James E. Gilliam.

Graham, K.A. (2003) "Coaching for friendship, eye to eye." *The Philadelphia Inquirer,* August.

Gray, C. (1994) *Comic Strip Conversations.* Jenison, MI: Jenison Public Schools.

Gray, C. (2000) *Writing Social Stories.* Arlington, TX: Future Horizons Inc.

Gray, S., Ruble, L. and Dalrymple, N. (1996) *Autism and Sexuality: A Guide for Instruction.* Bloomington, IN: Autism Society of Indiana.

Griffiths, D. (1999) *La sexualité des personnes présentant un trouble envahissant du développement.* Consortium de Services pour les Personnes ayant des Troubles Graves du Comportement. Conférence: Montréal.

Griffiths, D. (2000) "The case of Bruce." Presented at the Sixth Annual Sexuality Conference on Double Jeopardy, Welland and District Association for Community Living, Niagara Falls, Ontario, Canada.

Griffiths, D., Quinsey, V.L. and Hingsburger, D. (1989) *Changing Inappropriate Sexual Behavior.* Baltimore, MD: Paul H. Brookes.

Griffiths, D., Richards, D., Fedoroff, P. and Watson, S.L. (2002) *Ethical Dilemmas: Sexuality and Developmental Disability.* New York: NADD Press.

Hali, I. and Bernai, J. (1995) "Asperger's syndrome and violence: Correspondence." *British Journal of Psychiatry 166,* 262.

Hall, K. (2001) *Asperger Syndrome, the Universe and Everything.* London: Jessica Kingsley Publishers.

Haracopos, D. and Pedersen, L. (1999) *The Danish Report.* Kettering: Autism Independent UK.

Hatfield, E. (1984) "The danger of intimacy." In V.J. Derlaga (ed.) *Communication, Intimacy and Close Relationship.* Orlando, FL: Academic Press.

Health Canada and GlaxoSmithKline Inc., Government of Canada (2003) *Le PAXIL® ne doit pas être employé chez les enfants et les adolescents de moins de 18 ans.* www.hc-sc.gc.ca/english

Health Quebec, Government of Quebec (1991) *Enquête sociale et de santé auprès des enfants et adolescents Quebecois.* Quebec: Ministere de la Santé et des Services Sociaux du Québec.

Hedgcock, R. (2002) "Confessions of a borderline Aspie." Handout notes. Asperger Syndrome Support Network, Victoria, Australia.

Hellemans, H. (1996) "L'éducation sexuelle des adolescents autistes." Paper presented at the Project Caroline Conference: Bruxelles.

Hellemans, H. and Deboutte, D. (2002) "Autism spectrum disorders and sexuality." Conference: Melbourne World Autism Congress.

Hénault, I. (2000) "Plaidoyer pour l'ambiguïté sexuelle." *Guide ressources.* February.

Hénault, I. (2003) "The sexuality of adolescents with Asperger syndrome." In L. Holliday Willey (ed.) *Asperger Syndrome in Adolescence: Living with the Ups, the Downs, and Things In Between.* London: Jessica Kingsley Publishers.

Hénault, I. (2004) "Sexual relationships." In L.J. Baker and L.Welkowitz (eds) *Asperger's Syndrome: Intervening in Schools, Clinics, and Communities.* New Jersey: Lawrence Erlbaum Associates.

Hénault, I. and Attwood, T. (2002) *The Sexual Profile of Adults with Asperger Syndrome: The Need for Comprehension, Support and Education.* Melbourne: World Inaugural Autism Congress Publications.

Hénault, I., Forget, J. and Giroux, N. (2003) "Le développement d'habiletés sexuelles adaptatives chez des individus atteints d'Autisme de haut niveau ou du syndrome d'Asperger." Thèse présentée comme exigence partielle du doctorat en psychologie. Université du Québec à Montréal.

Hess, U. (1998) "L'intelligence émotionnelle." Course notes (PSY 4080). Montréal: Université du Québec à Montréal.

Hingsburger, D. (1993) *I Openers: Parents Ask Questions About Sexuality and Children with Developmental Disabilities.* Vancouver: Family Support Institute Press.

Hingsburger, D. (1995a) *Hand Made Love: A Guide for Teaching About Male Masturbation Through Understanding and Video.* Newmarket: Diverse City Press. *www.diverse-city.com*

Hingsburger, D. (1995b) *Just Say Know! Understanding and Reducing the Risk of Sexual Victimization of People with Developmental Disabilities.* Newmarket: Diverse City Press. *www.diverse-city.com*

Hingsburger, D. (1995c) *No! How! Understanding and Reducing the Risk of Sexual Victimization of People with Developmental Disabilities.* Video. Newmarket: Diverse City Press. *www.diverse-city.com*

Hingsburger, D. (1996) *Under Cover Dick: Teaching Men with Disabilities about Condom Use Through Understanding and Video.* Newmarket: Diverse City Press. *www.diverse-city.com*

Hingsburger, D. and Haar, S. (2000) *Finger Tips: Teaching Women with Disabilities about Masturbation Through Understanding and Video.* Newmarket: Diverse City Press. *www.diverse-city.com*

Holliday Willey, L. (1999) *Pretending to be Normal: Living with Asperger's Syndrome.* London: Jessica Kingsley Publishers.

Holliday Willey, L. (2001) *Asperger Syndrome in the Family: Redefining Normal.* London: Jessica Kingsley Publishers.

Howes, N. (1982) *Fully Human: A Program in Human Sexuality for the Developmentally Disabled.* Cambridge: Sun-Rose Associates, Black and White.

Howlin, P., Baron-Cohen, S. and Hadwin, J. (1999) *Teaching Children with Autism to Mind-read.* London: John Wiley.

Israel, G.E. and Tarver, D.E. (1997) *Transgender Care.* Philadelphia, PA: Temple University Press.

Jackson, L. (2002) *Freaks, Geeks and Asperger Syndrome: A User Guide to Adolescence.* London: Jessica Kingsley Publishers.

Jacobson, N.S. and Gurman, A.S. (1995) *Clinical Handbook of Couple Therapy.* New York: The Guilford Press.

Kaeser, F. and O'Neill, J. (1987) "Task analysed masturbation instruction for a profoundly mentally retarded adult male: A data based case study." *Sexuality and Disability 8,* 17–24.

Kanner, L. (1943) "Autistic disturbances of affective contact." *Nervous Child 2,* 217–250.

Keating, K. (1983) *The Hug Therapy Book.* Minneapolis, MN: CompCare Publishers.

Keating, K. (1994) *Le petit livre des gros câlins* (The Little Book of Big Hugs). Paris: Seuil.

Keesling, B. (1993) *Sexual Pleasure: Reaching New Heights of Sexual Arousal and Intimacy.* Alameda: Hunter House, Inc.

Kempton, W. (1993) *Socialization and Sexuality: A Comprehensive Guide.* Santa Barbara, CA: James Stanfield Company.

Kempton, W. (1999) *Life Horizons I and II.* Santa Barbara, CA: James Stanfield Company.

Klin, A., Volkmar, F.R. and Sparrow, S.S. (2000) *Asperger Syndrome.* New York: The Guilford Press.

Kohn, Y., Fahum, T. and Ratzoni, G. (1998) "Aggression and sexual offense in Asperger's syndrome." *Israel Journal of Psychiatry and Related Science 35,* 4, 293–9.

Konstantareas, M.M. and Lunsky, Y.J. (1997) "Sociosexual knowledge, experience, attitudes, and interests of individuals with autistic disorder and developmental delay." *Journal of Autism and Developmental Disorders* 27, 113–125.

L'Abate, L. and Sloan, S. (1984) "A workshop format to facilitate intimacy in married couples." *Family Relations* 33, 245–50.

Landen, M. and Rasmussen, P. (1997) "Gender identity disorder in a girl with autism: A case report." *European Child and Adolescent Psychiatry* 6, 170–3.

Laxer, G. and Tréhin, P. (2001) *Les troubles du comportement associés à l'autisme et aux autres handicaps mentaux.* Mougins: AFD.

Lazarus, A. (1976) *Multimodal Behavior Therapy.* New York: Springer.

Lemay, M. (1996) *La SexoTrousse.* Maniwaki: Pavillon du Parc.

Lieberman, A. and Melone, M.B. (1979) *Sexuality and Social Awareness.* Connecticut, CT: Benhaven Press.

Luiselli, J.K., Helfen, C.S., Pemberton, B.W. and Reisman, J. (1977) "The elimination of a child's in-class masturbation by overcorrection and reinforcement." *Journal of Behavioral Therapy and Experimental Psychiatry* 8, 201–4.

Margolin, G. (1982) "A social learning approach to intimacy." In M. Fisher and G. Stricker (ed.) *Intimacy.* New York: Plenum.

Marshburn, E.C. and Aman, M.G. (1992) "Factor validity and norms for the Aberrant Behavior Checklist in a community sample of children with mental retardation." *Journal of Autism and Developmental Disorders* 22, 357–73.

Masters, W.H. and Johnson, V.E. (1968) *Les réactions sexuelles.* Paris: Robert Laffont.

Masters, W.H. and Johnson, V.E. (1970) *Human Sexual Inadequacy.* Boston, MA: Little and Brown.

Mawson, D., Grounds, A. and Tantam, D. (1985) "Violence and Asperger's syndrome: A case study." *British Journal of Psychiatry 147,* 566–9.

Mayes, S.D., Calhoun, S.L. and Crites, D.L. (2001) "Does DSM-IV Asperger's disorder exist?" *Journal of Abnormal Child Psychology 29,* 3, 263–71.

McAdams, D.P. (1988) "Personal needs and personal relationships." In S.W. Duck (ed.) *Handbook of Personal Relationships: Theory, Research, and Intervention.* New York: John Wiley and Sons.

McCarthy, M. (1993) "Sexual experiences of women with learning difficulties in long-stay hospitals." *Sexuality and Disability 2,* 4, 277.

McCarthy, M. and Phil, B. (1996) "The sexual support needs of people with learning disabilities: A profile of those referred for sex education." *Sexuality and Disability 14,* 265–79.

McKee, L. and Blacklidge, V. (1986) *An Easy Guide for Caring Parents: Sexuality and Socialization.* Shasta-Diablo, CA: Planned Parenthood.

Melone, M.B. and Lettick, A.L. (1979) *Sex Education at Benhaven: Benhaven Then and Now.* Connecticut, CT: The Benhaven Press.

Miller, J.N. and Ozonoff, S. (2000) "The external validity of Asperger Disorder: Lack of evidence from the domain of neuropsychology." *Journal of Abnormal Psychology 109,* 2, 227–38.

Ministry of Health and Social Services (Gouvernement of Quebéc: Coordination Centre On AIDS) (1999) "Preventing AIDS and other STDs through sexuality education for students with intellectual impairments – compendium of teaching and learning activities geared to adapted curricula." *www.msss.gouv.qc.ca*

Moebius, M. (1998) "Gender identity disorder and psychosexual problems in children and adults: Book reviews." *Journal of the American Academy of Child and Adolescent Psychiatry,* March, 337.

Mukaddes, N.M. (2002) "Gender identity problems in autistic children." *Child: Care Health and Development,* *28,* 529–32.

Muskat, B. (2003) "Nonverbal learning disabilities and Asperger Syndrome: Enhancing socialization and emotional well-being." The Second National Conference on Asperger's Syndrome, Aspergers Society of Ontario.

National Information Center for Children and Youth with Disabilities (1992) "Sexuality education for children and youth with disabilities." *NICHCY News Digest 17,* 1–37.

Newport, J. and Newport, M. (2002) *Autism – Asperger's and Sexuality: Puberty and Beyond.* Arlington, TX: Future Horizons Inc.

Ouellet, R. and L'Abbé, Y. (1986) *Programme d'entraînement aux habiletés sociales.* Eastman: Éditions Behaviora.

Ouellet, R., Bandeira, M. and L'Abbé, Y. (1987) "L'entraînement aux habiletés sociales et la généralisation." *Revue de modification du comportement 17,* 76–94.

Ousley, O.Y. and Mesibov, G.B. (1991) "Sexual attitudes and knowledge of high-functioning adolescents and adults with autism." *Journal of Autism and Developmental Disorders 21,* 471–81.

Paradis, A.F. and Lafond, J. (1990) *La réponse sexuelle et ses perturbations.* Boucherville: Les Editions G. Vermette.

Poirier, N. (1998) "La théorie de l'esprit de l'enfant autiste." *Santé Mentale au Québec 23,* 1, 115–129.

Poirier, N. and Forget, J. (1998) "Les critères diagnostiques de l'autisme et du syndrome d'Asperger: Similitudes et différences." *Santé Mentale au Québec 23,* 1, 130–48.

Projet TRIP (1997) *Silence on SEX… Prime. Document Vidéo en Trois Volets.* Hôpital Rivière-des-Prairies: CECOM.

Robison, P.C., Conahan, F. and Brady, W. (1992) "Reducing self-injurious masturbation using a least intrusive model and adaptative equipment." *Sexuality and Disability 10,* 1, 43–55.

Rodman, K.E. (2003) *Asperger Syndrome and Adults… Is Anyone Listening? Essays and Poems by Spouses, Partners and Parents of Adults With Asperger Syndrome.* London: Jessica Kingsley Publishers.

Rosenberg, M. (2002) "Children with gender identity issues and their parents in individual and group treatment: Clinical perspectives." *Journal of the American Academy of Child and Adolescent Psychiatry,* May, 619–621.

Roy, J. (1996) "Comparaison entre les attitudes des intervenants travaillant auprès d'adolescents autistes et ceux travaillant auprès d'adolescents déficients intellectuellement à l'égard des comportements sexuels de ces jeunes." *Rapport d'Activités de Maîtrise en Sexologie.* Département de sexologie, Université du Québec à Montréal.

Ruble, L.A. and Dalrymple, J. (1993) "Social/sexual awareness of persons with autism: A parental perspective." *Archives of Sexual Behavior 22,* 229–40.

Schopler, E., Mesibov, G.B. and Kunce, L.J. (1998) *Asperger Syndrome or High-Functioning Autism?* New York: Plenum Press.

Scragg, P. and Shah, A. (1994) "Prevalence of Asperger's Syndrome in a secure hospital." *British Journal of Psychiatry 165,* 679–82.

Sexuality Information and Education Council of the US (1991) *Sexuality Education for People with Disabilities.* New York: SIECUS.

Sharper Image Design (1999) *Biotouch Interactive Mood Light. www.sharperimage.com*

Sheehan, S. (2002) "Consent for sexual relations." In D.M. Griffiths, D. Richards, P. Fedoroff and S.L. Watson (eds) *Ethical Dilemmas: Sexuality and Developmental Disability.* New York: NADD Press.

Slater-Walker, G. and Slater-Walker, C. (2002) *An Asperger Marriage.* London: Jessica Kingsley Publishers.

Smith Myles, B., Bock, S. and Simpson, R. (2000) *Asperger Syndrome Diagnostic Scale.* Austin, TX: Pro Ed.

Smith Myles, B. and Southwick, J. (1999) *Aspergers Syndrome and Difficult Moments: Practical Solutions for Tantrums, Rage, and Meltdowns.* Shawnee Mission, KS: Autism Asperger Publishing Company.

Smith Myles, B., Tapscott Cook, K., Miller, N.E., Rinner, L. and Robbins, L.A. (2000) *Asperger Syndrome and Sensory Issues.* Shawnee Mission, KS: AAPC.

Sofronoff, K. and Attwood, T. (2002) "A cognitive behaviour therapy intervention for anxiety in children with Asperger's Syndrome." *Good Autism Practice 4,* 228.

Soyner, R. and Desnoyers Hurley, A. (1990) "L'apprentissage des habiletés sociales." *Habilitative Mental Healthcare Newsletter 9,* 1, 1–5.

Stanford, A. (2002) *Asperger Syndrome and Long-Term Relationships.* London: Jessica Kingsley Publishers.

Stavis, P. and Walker-Hirsch, L.W. (1999) "Consent to sexual activity." In R.D. Dinerstein, S.S. Herr and J.L. O'Sullivan (eds) *A Guide to Consent.* Washington, DC: American Association on Mental Retardation.

Stoddart, K. (2003) "Young adults with AS: Benefiting from services and supports in the midst of transition." The Second National Conference on Asperger's Syndrome, Toronto: Aspergers Society of Ontario.

Stonehouse, M. (2002) *Stilted Rainbow: The Story of My Life on the Autistic Spectrum and a Gender Indentity Conflict.* Toronto: Martine Stonehouse.

Stonehouse, M. (2003) *Gender Identity Conflicts on the Autistic Spectrum and the Possible Co-Morbidity Between Them.* Toronto: Canadian–American Research Consortium on Autistic Spectrum Disorders.

Stonehouse, M. (forthcoming) *Stilted Rainbow – A Summary, Book of First Hand Accounts.*

Swisher, S. (1995) "Therapeutic interventions recommended for treatment of sexual addiction-compulsivity." *Sexual Addiction and Compulsivity 2,* 1, 31–9.

Szatmari, P., Bremner, R. and Nagy, J.N. (1989) "Asperger's syndrome: A review of clinical features." *Canadian Journal of Psychiatry 34,* 6, 554–60.

Team Asperger (2000) *Gaining Face.* Wisconsin, WN: Team Asperger.

Timmers, R.L., DuCharme, P. and Jacob, G. (1981) "Sexual knowledge, attitudes and behaviors of developmentally disabled adults living in a normalized apartment setting." *Sexuality and Disability 4,* 27–39.

Torisky, D. and Torisky, C. (1985) "Sex education and sexual awareness building for autistic children and youth: Some viewpoints and consideration." *Journal of Autism and Developmental Disorders 15,* 213–227.

Tréhin, C. (1999) *Les autistes de haut niveau et ceux atteints d'un syndrome d'Asperger.* Le Cannet: EDI Formation.

Tréhin, C. (2002) personal communication.

Tremblay, G., Desjardins, J. and Gagnon, J.P. (1993) *Programme de développement psychosexuel.* Ramaville, France: Eastman, Éditions Behaviora.

Tremblay, R., Aragon, A., Paunero, G., Suret, N. and Vidotto, M.C. (2001) *Guide d'éducation sexuelle à l'usage des professionnels, tome II.* Editions Eres.

Tremblay, R., Trombert, H., Lanacherie, O., Guinard, M., Dal Morro, M. and Beslot, J. (1998) *Guide d'éducation sexuelle à l'usage des professionnels tome I.* Editions Eres.

University of Iowa (2003) *Virtual Hospital.* Department of Psychiatry. *www.vh.org.*

Van Bourgondien, M., Reichle, N.C. and Palmer, A. (1997) "Sexual behavior in adults with autism." *Journal of Autism and Developmental Disorders 27,* 2, 113–25.

Walker-Hirsch, L. and Champagne, M.P. (1986) *Circles I, II and III.* Santa Barbara, CA: James Stanfield Company.

Weiss, R.S. (1973) *Loneliness: The Experience of Emotional and Social Isolation.* Cambridge, MA: MIT Press.

WHO (World Health Organization) (1993) *International Classification of Diseases, Tenth Revision* (ICD-10). Geneva: WHO.

Wing, L. (1981) "Asperger's Syndrome: A clinical account." *Psychological Medicine 11*, 115–30.

Wing, L. (1991) "The relationship between Asperger's Syndrome and Kanner's autism." In U. Frith (ed.) *Autism and Asperger Syndrome.* New York: Cambridge University Press.

Young, E. (2001) "A look at theory of mind." *The New Scientist 29*, March.

Videos

Hingsburger, D. (1995) *No! How!!! Understanding and Reducing the Risk of Sexual Victimisation of People with Developmental Disabilities.* Video. Newmarket: Diverse City Press. www.diverse.city.com

Hingsburger, D. (1995) *Hand Made Love: A Guide for Teaching About Male Masturbation Through Understanding and Video.* Newmarket: Diverse City Press. *www.diverse-city.com*

Hingsburger, D. (1996) *Under Cover Dick: Teaching Men with Disabilities about Condom Use Through Understanding and Video.* Newmarket: Diverse City Press. *www.diverse-city.com*

Hingsburger, D. and Haar, S. (2000) *Finger Tips: Teaching Women with Disabilities about Masturbation Through Understanding and Video.* Newmarket: Diverse City Press. *www.diverse-city.com*

Internet resources

FAAAS organization (couples and Asperger families): *www.faaas.org*

National Autistic Society: *www.nas.org.uk*

Alcohol and young people

Government of Quebec, Health and Social Services: http://ftp.msss.gouv.qc.ca/publications/acrobat/f/documentation/2001/01-812-f-pdf

Interpersonal relationships and violence

Making Waves programme: *www.mwaves.org*

Medication

Virtual Hospital: *www.vh.org*

Sexuality

Autism Independent UK, United Kingdom: *www.autismuk.com/index9sub.htm*

NICHCY – National Dissemination Center for Children with Disabilities, Washington, DC: *www.nichcy.org*

Calgary Birth Control Association: *www.cbca.ab.ca*

Family Planning Queensland: *www.fpq.com.au*

Tools and programmes

Biofeedback GSR Biotouch Moodlight: *www.sharperimage.com*

Gaining Face, software on emotions: *http://www.ccoder.com/GainingFace*

Subject index

oestrogen 21
    see also hormones, sex
oral contraceptives 25
    see also contraception
orgasm 35, 128
Other Half of Asperger Syndrome, The
    (Aston) 96
ovary 129, 133
    functions of 34
ovum 129, 133
    functions of 34

paedophilia 55, 58, 62
PDD *see* pervasive developmental
    disorder
peer behaviour, imitation of
    27–8, 44
penis 23, 129, 131
    functions of 34
Penis Book, The (Cohen) 23
periods 21
personal hygiene 21, 23–4
pervasive developmental disorder
    (PDD) 15, 16, 43, 48, 87,
    101, 102, 184
physiological aspects of sexuality
    125–34
Positive Symptom Distress Index
    (PSDI) 184
Pretending to be Normal (Holliday
    Willey) 15
prevention, of STDs 144–50
    see also contraception
progesterone 21, 25
    see also sex hormones

*Programme d'éducation à la vie
    affective, amoureuse et sexuelle*
    (Desaulniers) 102
Programme d'éducation sexuelle
    (Durocher & Fortier) 102–3
promiscuity 48
prostate 129, 131
    functions of 34
puberty
    boys 23–4
    changes, accepting 24–5
    gender identity conflict 84,
        87, 88
    girls 21–3
    personal hygiene 21, 23–4
    physical changes 19

sexual education, need for
    19–21
    Workshop 4 126, 127
public/private behaviour,
    boundaries between 32, 43–4,
    57, 171

refractory period 128
rejection, feelings of 28–9
relaxation techniques 71
repression of sexual urges 43
retrograde ejaculation 41
    see also epididimitis;
        masturbation,
        problematic
risky sexual behaviours 160
Ritalin, side effects 42
romantic relationships, abuse in
    174–8

sado-masochistic behaviour 79
schizophrenia 17
scrotum 129, 131
    functions of 134
secondary sexual characteristics
    19
segregation, sexual 30–1
self-esteem 28–30, 65
self-image 27–8, 81–2
self-mutilation 45
sensate focus 99, 100
senses, and sexuality 17, 137–8,
    141
    see also hypersensitivity;
        hyposensitivity
Sex for One: The Joy of Selfloving
    (Dodson) 37
Sexo Trousse (Lemay) 102, 142
Sexoholics Anonymous 55
sexual abstinence 25
sexual abuse *see* abuse, sexual
sexual assault *see* assault, sexual
sexual behaviours
    studies of 32
    see also inappropriate sexual
        behaviours
sexual desire *see* desire, sexual
sexual development, factors
    affecting 30–1
sexual intimacy
    commitment 99
    erogenous zones 97–8

foreplay 98, 99
sensate focus exercise 99,
    100
sexual enrichment
    programme 99
sexual script 99
tactile sensitivities 98–9
sexual knowledge questionnaire
    30
sexual orientation
    ambisexuality 81–2
    asexuality 80
    and autism/AS diagnosis
        82
    bisexuality 79, 80, 82
    "effeminate" traits 81
    homophobia questionnaire
        157–8
    image, projection of 81–2
    sexual preference 79–80
    support groups 82–3
    Workshop 8 153–8
    see also gender identity;
        homosexuality
sexual profile, of adults with AS
    affect 187
    attitudes 188
    body image 186, 189, 190
    desire 188, 189
    DSFI, use of 183, 184
    experiences 186, 189,
        190–1
    fantasies 189–90
    general satisfaction 188
    information 187
    satisfaction 187–8, 190
    sexual roles 189
    sociosexual skills, lack of
        183
    study participants 183–4
    study results 184–5
    symptoms 186
sexual response cycle 34, 128
sexually transmitted diseases *see*
    HIV/STDs
social circles 175
social influences 27–30
social isolation 17, 28–9, 41
social skills
    affectionate behaviour
        67–8
    automatic thoughts 71–4
    "breaking the ice" 65
    communication 66, 68–70

Author index

Abelson, A.G. 86
Adolphs, R. 74
Alarie, P. 41
Aman, M.G. 106
American Psychiatric Association
    (APA) 16
Aquilla, P. 40
Arturo Silva, J. 62
Asperger, H. 15
Asperweb France 39
Aston, M.C. 15, 31, 32, 96
Attwood, T. 12, 15–16, 17, 18,
    29, 30, 31, 45, 59, 64, 66, 68,
    78, 96, 101, 105, 106,
    183–92

Barbach, L. 99
Baron-Cohen, S. 17, 70, 74, 102,
    104, 105, 142, 179, 184
Basso, M.J. 20
Beaudoin, L. 140
Beaudry, M. 64, 68–9
Bernai, J. 61
Binet, A. 79
Bock, S. 18
Boisvert, J.-M. 64, 68–9
Bradley, S.J. 83, 84, 86
Bremner, R. 16
Brent, E. 74

Carnes, P. 54–5
Champagne, L.E. 175
Channon, S. 74, 105
Chipouras, S. 101, 190
Cohen, J. 23
Cohen-Kettenis, P.T. 86
Coleman, E. 55
Collacott, R.A. 61
Cooper, S.A. 61
Curnoe, S. 62

Dalrymple, N. 32, 43, 101
de Brosses, C. 79
De Myer, M.K. 32, 46

Deboutte, D. 32, 37, 39, 46, 63
Derogatis, L.R. 106, 183, 184
Desaulniers, M.P. 39, 102
Desnoyers Hurley, A. 102, 104
Dodson, B. 37
Dorais, M. 76–7
Dubé, L. 90
Durocher, L. 26, 30, 102–3, 106,
    169

Ehlers, S. 17, 61
Erickson, E.H. 90

Fahum, T. 61
Family Planning Queensland 21,
    22, 23, 26, 101
Ferrari, M. 62
Foreman, J. 97
Forget, J. 30
Fortier, M. 26, 30, 102–3, 106,
    169
Frith, U. 15

Gale, T. 83, 84
Gallucci, G. 86
Ghaziuddin, M. 61
Gillberg, C. 16, 17, 19, 39, 46,
    60, 61
Giroux, N. 30
Graham, K.A. 67
Gray, C. 18, 49, 66, 78, 106,
    179
Gray, S. 32, 43, 101
Griffiths, D. 30, 31, 41, 43, 44,
    50, 62, 101, 105, 190
Grounds, A. 61
Gurman, A.S. 99

Haar, S. 34
Hackerman, F. 86
Hadwin, J. 74
Hali, I. 61
Haracopos, D. 18, 19, 32, 34, 37,
    57, 101, 103, 190
Hatfield, E. 90
Hedgecock, R. 95
Hellemans, H. 19, 32, 37, 39, 46,
    190

Hénault, I. 30, 32, 46, 66, 70,
    77, 100, 103, 105, 106,
    183–92
Hess, U. 74
Hingsburger, D. 19, 30, 31, 33,
    34, 43, 50, 59, 101, 146, 168,
    190
Holliday Willey, L. 15
Howlin, P. 74

Israel, G.E. 80, 83, 84, 85, 86

Jackson, L. 65
Jacobson, N.S. 99
Johnson, V.E. 34, 37, 57, 99,
    100, 128

Kaeser, F. 101
Kanner, L.
Keating, K. 67
Keesling, B. 99
Kempton, W. 18, 20, 25, 32, 39,
    101, 102, 103, 190
Klin, A. 15, 17
Kohn, Y. 61
Konstantareas, M.M. 37
Kunce, L.J. 16

L'Abate, L. 95
L'Abbé, Y. 67, 102
Lafond, J. 99
Landen, M. 86
Langevin, R. 62
Laxer, G. 41
Lazarus, A. 72–3
Lemay, M. 69, 102, 142
Leong, G. 62
Levenson, R.W. 97
Lunsky, Y.J. 37

Margolin, G. 95
Masters, W.H. 34, 37, 57, 99,
    100, 128
Mawson, D. 61
McAdams, D.P. 90
McCarthy, M. 48
Melisaratos, N. 106, 183, 184
Mesibov, G.B. 16, 19, 32, 39